TREATING ABUSED ADOLESCENTS

About the Author

Eliana Gil, Ph.D., is a licensed marriage, family, and child counselor who specializes in the treatment of abused children and adolescents and their families, as well as adult survivors. She is director of the Center for Advanced Clinical Development, Springfield, Virginia, and has a private practice in Rockville, Maryland. She is a registered play therapy supervisor and has written numerous books on treatment of children, including *The Healing Power of Play: Working with Abused Children* and *Play in Family Therapy*. Dr. Gil is an adjunct faculty member of the Virginia Tech University where she teaches family and play therapy courses. She serves on the board of directors of both the American Professional Society on the Abuse of Children and the National Resource Center on Child Sexual Abuse.

Treating
Abused Adolescents

ELIANA GIL

THE GUILFORD PRESS
New York London

© 1996 The Guilford Press
A Division of Guilford Publications, Inc.
72 Spring Street, New York, NY 10012

Printed in the United States of America

This book is printed on acid-free paper.

Last digit is print number: 9 8 7 6 5

Library of Congress Cataloging-in-Publication Data
Gil, Eliana
    Treating abused adolescents / Eliana Gil.
      p. cm.
    Includes bibliographical references and index.
    ISBN 1-57230-114-7.–ISBN 1-57230-115-5 (pbk.)
    1. Abused teenagers. 2. Adolescent psychotherapy.
  I. Title.
RJ507.A29G553 1996
616.85′82239′00835–dc20   96-12550
                                                            CIP

To Kiddo

*Thank you for allowing me to be there
on the occasion of your transition
from childhood. I will never forget you,
what we shared, and what we
learned from each other.*

Acknowledgments

I would like to take this opportunity to publicly acknowledge Kathy Baxter, executive director of the San Francisco Child Abuse Council, and Lorraine Heath, administrative assistant to the Council. In spite of the fact that there is now a great geographical distance between us, I still regard the Council as my homebase – a place in which I feel unconditional support and positive regard. It's where I first developed an interest in this field, and where I was allowed to undertake many significant and valuable projects. I was very fortunate that Kathy Baxter was my boss when I decided it was possible and desirable for me to pursue my education. In any other setting, I am convinced, I would not have found the generosity and support that Kathy provided. She created an unrestricted environment in which I came to believe that I could do anything I set my mind to do. She encouraged me, pushed me, stimulated me, and gave me the freedom to design and implement many ideas that taught me immeasurable lessons. The more I learn, the more I appreciate Kathy's amazing trust and belief in me. Deep in my heart I know that without her I would not have imagined, or striven for, more. I am forever in her debt for this, as well as the fact that she has always been, and continues to be, my unwavering champion. For what I recognize as a long term friendship, I am grateful. I also thank Lorraine Heath, my rock of Gibraltar throughout many tough years of trying to balance work, family, and school. Lorraine kept up my spirits, dropped everything to chit-chat with me and encourage me when I felt down. Lorraine is a remarkable woman, mother, and "worker bee," whom I respect immensely and care for a great deal. We've shared a lot together, including joys, sorrows, stressful and exciting times, and mutual interests. I am fortunate to have her as a friend.

Karren Campbell, a psychology doctoral student at the University of Maryland, researched and coauthored Chapter Two.

Turning to the production of this book, I give special thanks to Rochelle Serwator of Guilford Press for her respectful and creative help. She gave numerous concrete suggestions when I encountered obstacles in writing, and she encouraged and supported me most graciously. It has been a pleasure to have her thoughtful and astute guidance.

I have made every effort to protect my clients' confidentiality by altering identifying information such as gender and age, as well as providing clinical material gleaned from a compilation of cases. In most cases where dialogues are transcribed verbatim, clients have reviewed transcripts and provided written permission to reproduce specific segments of our therapeutic conversations (the group therapy session was constructed from memory and is not transcribed verbatim).

Contents

TREATING ABUSED ADOLESCENTS

CHAPTER ONE

Adolescence and Abuse: An Overview

Jennifer was referred to me shortly after giving birth to her daughter, Janine. Jennifer was 13 years old, with a look of fear and excitement in her eyes. She clung to her infant desperately and begged for reassurance that she would be allowed to keep the baby. She was living with a foster mother who was willing to care for both Jennifer and Janine; this was Jennifer's seventh foster placement.

Jennifer had been sexually abused by her mother's boyfriend when she was 2 years of age. The sexual abuse was extensive, and she required medical hospitalization for a sexually transmitted disease. She was removed from her mother's care and placed in an emergency foster home for a period of time. After the court terminated the parental rights of Jennifer's mother, she was transferred to a foster/adoptive home. The adoption was almost completed when the adoptive mother became physically ill and was no longer able to care for Jennifer, now an active 4-year-old. Jennifer considered this woman her mother and remembered being carried away from her home in tears. She then moved to three more foster homes in the next 6 years and did not allow herself to care for the people she lived with. At age 10, she ran away and lived "on the street" for approximately 9 months. She was taken to a hospital with pneumonia and released to the authorities, who once again placed her in a foster home. She got into fights at school, hung out with the "drug crowd," and cut school a lot. At age 11, she ran away again and was picked up for prostitution. She was sent to yet another foster home and this time seemed to respond well to the foster mother, who made concerted efforts to spend time with her and talk with her. Jennifer stayed in this foster home until she ran away with her boyfriend, a 22-year-old street peddler. After 8 months, her boyfriend "dumped" her and got a new girlfriend. Jennifer was again referred to protective services when she was picked up for panhandling. A medical examination revealed her to be 4 months pregnant, and she was returned to her former foster parent at her request.

Jennifer pleaded with me for a chance to love and take care of her baby. "She and I belong to each other," she stated. "No one is gonna love her like I can, and no one cares about me like she does." She was absolutely compelling and heartbreaking as she grasped her child tightly to her. "We belong to each other," she repeated. "I'll never let anything hurt her. I'll make sure she has everything she needs. I can do it – I want it."

Jennifer remained in her foster placement beyond the age of majority. Her foster mother, Glenna, became the parent she had never known; the three of them became a family, with baby Janine calling Glenna "Granny." Giving birth to Janine gave Jennifer a sense of identity and purpose. She had been unable to find the motivation to forge ahead on her own behalf, but she was adamant that she would succeed for her child in order to give her the kind of life she herself had never known. Although this type of rationale appears with regularity in work with teen mothers, in Jennifer's case it did not backfire, as it does with many other youngsters. Jennifer's motivation was fueled by her own sense of maternal deprivation, coupled with the fact that she had fortunately been able to receive love from and give love to her foster mother, Glenna. This positive relationship with Glenna was probably what gave her a model to follow – someone who could provide consistency and strength, in spite of the hard work and patience required.

Jennifer had suffered severe deprivation and loss as a child. She never knew her father; she was sexually abused as a toddler; and then her mother's inability or unwillingness to care for her resulted in termination of parental rights. Another early attachment to a potential adoptive home had been terminated abruptly when the adoptive mother became ill (and later died). Clearly, Jennifer had lacked parental nurturing and guidance, and had never developed a sense of belonging. Her first serious romantic attachment also resulted in disappointment and pain as she was unceremoniously replaced.

In spite of the overwhelming problems she encountered in her childhood, Jennifer emerged a strong and determined youngster, who elicited and returned her foster mother's care and concern. When she learned of her pregnancy she felt "reborn," as if now she had a chance to give to someone else what she had not been given.

This youngster's resiliency is remarkable and is a tribute to the human instinct to thrive and survive in the face of great obstacles. And yet the same hardships that Jennifer faced challenge thousands of youngsters, not all of whom are able to find the inner resources, engage in a positive relationship with another, or find the motivation to persevere.

Child abuse and neglect are powerful deterrents to healthy growth and development. How some children find the strength or the willingness to keep trying boggles the mind. And yet many of us are in a position to have therapeutic relationships with adolescents who have been abused, and we have an opportunity to contribute something to their development – at the very least, a new experience about the possible rewards of human interactions.

This book is about adolescents with histories of current or past abuse. It describes how the lessons of abuse affect them, and how they "act out" in attempts to get attention and help. It also describes how we can help, and how helping adolescents is often difficult because they fight our best efforts. Their resistance, however, must be understood in the context of safety: As long as they continue to feel unsafe and distrustful, they will stay on guard. When they feel cared about, they may feel more frightened than ever. Finally, when they recognize that we won't be scared away or discouraged, they may give us the opportunity and privilege to be of assistance. A recent *Time* magazine article ("Generation Excluded," 1995) discusses the Carnegie Council on Adolescent Development's (1995) report entitled *Great Transitions,* and notes a "disturbing portrait of

America as a dismissive and preoccupied parent, a country trying to wish away the troubles of its teenagers" (p. 86). The report shows that it is at the phase of adolescence that parental involvement in school activities drops off. One of the report's prescriptions is for health professionals to increase their efforts to educate and treat adolescents. I think it behooves us all to become better informed and more involved in assisting adolescents who experience an array of concerns: some emerging during adolescence and others experienced during childhood and related to parental maltreatment or underinvolvement, lack of guidance and structure, family conflict, or family dysfunction.

Before I go on to examine the extent and impact of abuse of adolescents, it is useful to consider what we mean by "adolescence" itself, as well as some of the assumptions we all make about adolescents.

WHAT IS ADOLESCENCE?

The development of "adolescence" has political and social roots that are only a little over 100 years old (M. A. Straus, 1994). At one time (before the period spanning the 1880s to 1920s), individuals who would now be considered adolescents were expected to work as soon as they were strong enough physically (Katz, 1981). They contributed much to the economic and social stability of their families (M. A. Straus, 1994). Marriages were frequently arranged, and what one's family needed determined one's future (Gillis, 1981).

The Industrial Revolution (M. A. Straus, 1994) resulted in considerable social policy reformations: The juvenile and adult justice systems were separated, high school was made compulsory, and the first child labor laws were passed (Janus, McCormack, Burgess, & Hartman, 1987; M. A. Straus, 1994). It also increased the need to be educated in order to be economically successful (Barker, 1990; Janus et al., 1987). In addition, new types of industrial jobs made the labor market smaller; in order to prevent teenagers from competing with adults for jobs, childhood was extended. People therefore entered the work force later in life because they stayed in school longer. This change precipitated the invention of the enticing concept of "adolescence" (Barker, 1990; Janus et al., 1987; M. A. Straus, 1994). Once the concept was defined, there was a need to create special programs and institutions for this newly created age group.

Demographic changes and myths about "Americanism" also sustained the significance of adolescence (M. A. Straus, 1994). Parents and communities focused on providing education to ensure later success for their children (Barker, 1990; Janus et al., 1987). Also, the humanitarian laws mentioned above reinforced the extension of adolescence: Less emphasis was placed on the customary periods of apprenticeship and more on youngsters' development. This shift in focus helped shape today's adaptive alliance between parents and children, which allows for successful growth and transition into young adult life (Janus et al., 1987).

"Adolescence" is generally defined as the period of life between the ages of 10 and 21 (Flannery, Torquati, & Lindemeier, 1994), though slight variations are frequently reported. For the purposes of this book, "adolescents" are defined as young persons between the ages of 13 and 18. Those aged 17 and under are legally regarded as minors; 18-year-olds are legally regarded as adults.

Adolescence is a compelling phase of life. It is alternately described as exciting, chaotic, tumultuous, unsettling, risky, conflictual, joyous, and momentous. Adolescents as a group can be tremendously creative, compassionate, challenging, provocative, responsible, reckless, carefree, studious, focused, hostile, violent, passive–aggressive, or calm and peaceful. The range of adolescent behaviors is vast, and yet various assumptions often define our expectations of this age group.

SOME ASSUMPTIONS ABOUT ADOLESCENTS

On occasion, I have heard reports of television and newspaper surveys that indicate that adults become frightened when they see groups of adolescents, fearing assaults, burglaries, or other dangerous behaviors; apparently these fears are exacerbated when youngsters are black, Hispanic, or Asian. Adults also expect adolescents to be challenging or demanding, or to defy authority. Often clinicians hesitate to take referrals of adolescents, citing reasons such as personal discomfort, or pessimism about what can be accomplished.

Another assumption about adolescence is that it is always disordered, difficult, perilous, tumultuous, and painful for youngsters; however, many adults view their own adolescence as "the best years of their lives." Is adolescent turmoil fact or fiction?

Adolescents seemingly find and lose themselves at the same time (Janus et al., 1987). Turmoil proponents say that profound disruption of one's personality organization is normal at this stage and causes mood swings, unpredictable behavior, thought confusion, and rebelliousness. They believe that adolescents are unable to grow into mature, mentally healthy adults without it. According to psychoanalytic theory, a weakened ego combined with strong instinctual drives prevents teenagers from being balanced and harmonious: Their drives may lead them into delinquency, but repression of their drives leads to phobias and depression. M. B. Straus (1994) notes that being "normal" during adolescence is in fact abnormal. Similarly, Erikson (1963) believed that turmoil is requisite for normal development. He introduced the term "identity crisis," noting that expected fluctuations of ego strength cause increased conflicts, which lead to confusion, role struggles, and subsequent identity formation.

Many others disagree with the idea that turmoil is an expected and unavoidable aspect of adolescence. M. B. Straus (1994) states that the struggle between parents and their children is conventional, but not necessary. Individual development can take many routes, some of which are smooth while others are more turbulent, but not completely full of emotional turmoil. Each teenager faces and handles these challenges in different ways.

Experimental research does not support controversial turmoil theories. Findings suggest that most adolescents feel happy, strong, and self-confident, and do not have serious conflicts with their parents (Hill, 1993; M. B. Straus, 1994). Only 20% report problems with social and personal areas (Offer & Sabshin, 1984), and only one in five families experience frequent disputes (Hill, 1993). Only 20% of nonpatient adolescents report turmoil severe enough for them to run away from home (Janus et al., 1987). The clinical samples that Erikson (1963) used in formulating the identity crisis theory, although convenient, were biased and did not represent the typical adolescent (M. B. Straus, 1994).

Though adolescents and their parents may frequently disagree about hairstyles, clothing, and curfews, serious conflicts are rare, and typically occur when adolescents suffer from a psychiatric disorder. It is not unusual for adolescents to experience some inner turmoil, characterized by misery or self-deprecation, but not all adolescents experience these emotions, and some manifestations are mild (Rutter, Graham, Chadwick, & Yule, 1976). As for the effects of so-called "raging" hormones and emotions on behavior, these not only are small but are influenced by nonhormonal factors, such as gender, temperament, age, pubertal status, and pubertal timing (Buchanan, Eccles, & Becker, 1992, as cited in Flannery et al., 1994).

In short, not all adolescents have major identity crises; however, not all families are carefree (M. B. Straus, 1994). In order to avoid subscribing to damaging myths about adolescent turmoil, clinicians must consider the normal range of development in context. When adolescent development is assessed, it is advisable to use a broad lens to consider all the aspects of development that undergo changes during this life stage (see Chapter Two for a full discussion of these).

UNDERSTANDING THE BASIC NEEDS OF ADOLESCENTS

When I have attended lectures about adolescent development or adolescent issues, it is my impression that people often restrict their discussions to a particular dimension of adolescent development, such as cognitive or personality development. Only recently have I seen efforts to consider adolescence in a broader context that includes physical, cognitive, emotional (attachment), personality, moral, sexual, and spiritual development (Newton, 1995). There is a great deal of impetus for growth and change during this stage of life, and youngsters are negotiating often opposing drives (e.g., biological development and moral development).

Clinicians must examine the various developmental dimensions that are in flux during this period, as well as identifying obstacles to development in specific dimensions. For example, some emotions, behaviors, and thought processes, though seemingly inappropriate, may be developmentally typical; other behaviors, emotions, and thought processes may be developmentally inappropriate.

Schrodt and Fitzgerald (1987) have documented several normal "problems" in dealing with adolescents. They may distort time, have an exaggerated sense of loyalty to their peers, mistrust adults, be extremely self-conscious, and periodically suspend logic. They may also have insufficient motivation for change, lack persistence, and have difficulty verbalizing their concerns.

Unless we understand the developmental needs of adolescents, what we see and hear from them will be difficult to understand (Barker, 1990). Understanding the typical progression of phases and tasks in adolescence serves therapists well in many domains (Corder, 1994); most notably, it provides them with identifiable and feasible goals when they are devising treatment plans. Therapists may also become more empathetic and patient in dealing with adolescents when they see their behavior in a larger context.

Viewing an adolescent in the context of his or her life stage may also prevent misunderstandings and miscommunications between the therapist and the adolescent, which might hinder the therapeutic process or lead the adolescent to terminate therapy. For example, periods of developmental challenges may cause maladaptive responses in the clinical setting (Forehand & Wierson, 1993). Developmental issues affect perception, conceptualization, and interpersonal styles (Bierman & Schwartz, 1986, as cited in Barker, 1990).

Finally, it is not only the adolescent's developmental issues that need attention. Therapists must also understand their own difficulties with their developmental tasks as adolescents before they begin to conduct therapy with adolescents (Corder, 1994).

UNDERSTANDING OBSTACLES
TO ADOLESCENT DEVELOPMENT

The obstacles to a gradual and even developmental process are many. When working with adolescents with specific symptoms, we may be able to surmise the origin of their problems. For example, when Walsh and Rosen (1988) studied 52 adolescent self-mutilators in treatment settings, they found that their backgrounds were replete with aversive events, such as sexual abuse, significant loss, and conflict with peers. Indeed, they found that a history of sexual abuse was the most useful in discriminating between mutilators who had been suicidal and those who had not.

Juveniles who sexually molest others have frequent histories either of parental loss or of family dysfunctions that are likely to affect child development, such as parent's violence against either the spouse or the children, parental substance abuse, and parents' experience of physical and sexual abuse in their own childhoods (Gil & Johnson, 1993; Ryan, 1991; Steen & Monnette, 1989). In fact, I have often heard informal reports from juvenile correctional institution personnel, which estimate that 90% of the youths referred to their program have histories of parental abuse or neglect.

It stands to reason, therefore, that youths undergoing specific types of stresses – such as abuse or neglect; physical illness; parental death, loss, or divorce; birth of siblings; and parent/caretaker dysfunction – require careful attention and support. Obviously, these circumstances may overload an already full schedule of difficult demands placed on them by the normal developmental process. Coping with external stressors overtaxes the available resources allocated for developmental tasks. Some adolescents appear to dig deeper, developing new resources; others are fortunate enough to seek out and obtain assistance from others in their environment, including adults in position of authority, religious or spiritual leaders, peers, or extended family members; still others derive support from formal and informal therapies and other means of survival, such as music, literature, sports, or academics. Adolescents who (for whatever reason) are unable to do any of these things may have severe difficulties coping with a range of normative or non-normative stressors.

As clinicians, our tasks in working with adolescents are not unlike those in working with younger children: to remove obstacles to developmental growth, and to attempt to ensure environmental conditions that will promote and enhance the developmental process. Many adolescents' problems occur because they have had difficulty in completing a developmental task (Barker, 1990). In work with children of any age, understanding family and social pressures or supports is pivotal to understanding the youngsters' difficulties and helping them to develop more reliable and secure support systems.

THE EXTENT OF ADOLESCENT ABUSE

In 1986, the American Humane Association's *Highlights of Official Child Neglect and Abuse Reporting* documented that of approximately 1.7 million cases of child maltreatment, 24% involved youths between 12 and 17 years of age. In 1978, the American Humane Association's report, *National Analysis of Official Child Abuse and Neglect Reporting,* demonstrated that adolescents aged 12–17 were the reported victims of 27.3% of all abuse/neglect cases. Using secondary data from the 1988 Study of National Incidence and Prevalence of Child Abuse and Neglect, Powers and Eckenrode (1992) also found that adolescents constituted a large proportion of all estimated cases of maltreatment; that more adolescents were more often emotionally abused than young children; that adolescent maltreatment more often involved female victims; and that more adolescent females experienced physical abuse than males.

According to a more recent incidence study (U.S. Department of Health and Human Services, 1995), almost 2 million reports of child abuse and neglect were received by child protective service agencies and referred for investigation in 1993. Nearly half of the victims of maltreatment (49%) suffered from neglect; 24% were physically abused; and 14% were sexually abused. Adolescents accounted for a lower percentage of reported victims than younger children did: 51% of victims were 7 years of age or younger, and 26% were 3 years of age or younger, whereas 20% were 13–18 years old (teenagers). The 1993 data regarding age were similar to those found in the previous 4 years of data collection. Fifty-one percent of the victims were female, and 45% were male; 54% were European-American, 25% African-American, and 9% Hispanic.

In a study of nonclinical and unreported adolescents totaling 3,998 students (Hibbard, Ingersoll, & Orr, 1990), 20% reported some form of physical or sexual abuse, with more girls than boys reporting sexual abuse. Although some problem behaviors were common among all adolescents, higher emotional and behavioral risk scores were confirmed among abused adolescents.

The true incidence of adolescent abuse may far exceed the documented statistics, for a number of reasons. Barth and Derezotes (1990) state that "the extent to which under reporting influences our estimate of the incidence of physical abuse, sexual abuse, neglect, and psychological maltreatment in adolescence is unknown" (p. 3). The actual *incidence* of adolescent maltreatment may not be lower than that of child maltreatment, but the *reporting* of it may, because of changed public perceptions of risk as children mature. Adolescents are often seen as having an increased ability to fight, run away, or otherwise fend off abuse. Moreover, there may be a pervasive belief that adolescents deserve the punishments they receive or that they can sustain physical punishment without damage. Finally, teenagers are often viewed more as potential victimizers than as potential victims, in spite of reports from the National Crime Survey and Uniform Crime Reports showing that teenagers are at substantially higher risk than their elders for all crimes except homicide (Moone, 1994), and that they are often targeted for stranger abduction (Finkelhor, Hotaling, & Sedlak, 1990).

TYPES OF ADOLESCENT ABUSE

"Child abuse" is a generic term for child maltreatment; it encompasses specific types of abuse as defined by law. Although reporting statutes vary from state to state, and the wording of definitions is also diverse, I quote the following formal definitions from the U.S. Department of Health and Human Services (1995):

> Maltreatment – An action or failure to act by a parent, caretaker, or other person, as defined under State law, having caused or allowed to cause physical abuse, neglect, medical neglect, sexual abuse, or emotional abuse harm, or risk of harm to a child. (p. B-4)

> Medical neglect – The harm by a caretaker to a child's health due to failure to provide for appropriate health care of the child, although financially able to do so, or offered financial or other means to do so. May include perinatal exposure to drugs. (p. B-4)

> Neglect or deprivation of necessities – A type of maltreatment that refers to the failure to provide needed, age-appropriate care, although financially able to do so, or offered other financial or other means to do so. (p. B-5)

> Physical abuse – A type of maltreatment that refers to physical acts that caused or could have caused physical injury of the child. (p. B-5)

> Psychological or emotional maltreatment – A type of maltreatment that refers to acts or omissions, other than physical abuse or sexual abuse, that caused, or could have caused, conduct, cognitive, affective or other mental disorders, such as emotional neglect, psychological abuse, mental injury, etc. (p. B-5)

> Sexual abuse – A type of maltreatment that refers to the involvement of the child in sexual activity to provide sexual gratification or financial benefit to the perpetrator, including contacts for sexual purposes, prostitution, pornography, exposure, or other sexually exploitative activities. (p. B-6)

Adolescents may be victimized in any of the above-mentioned ways. Moreover, some are victims of several types of abuse, and these youngsters may suffer greater consequences. In a study comparing physically and sexually abused adolescent inpatients, Hart, Mader, Griffith, and deMendonca (1989) found that adolescents who had been both physically and sexually abused displayed more drug abuse, reported more symptoms of distress, had more interpersonal problems, exhibited lower self-esteem, and engaged in more self-destructive behaviors.

There is ongoing discussion about the likelihood of youngsters' being more vulnerable to one or another type of abuse, based on their age and developmental needs. Finkelhor and Dziuba-Leatherman (1994) have devised a "dependency continuum for child victimization types," noting that "the main status characteristic of childhood is its condition of dependency, which is a function, at least in part, of social and psychological immaturity" (p. 177). They claim that it is the *violation* of the dependency status that results in forms of victimization: Physical neglect can only occur with a dependent person; family abduction is a dependency-specific victimization involving the removal of a child from a caretaker. Other forms of victimization, defined without reference to dependency status, exist for both adults and children (e.g., stranger abduction or homicide). Sexual abuse, according to Finkelhor and Dziuba-Leatherman, can occur with or without dependency-related status. Finkelhor (1995) states that sexual maturation makes children (especially girls) more vulnerable to sexually motivated crimes. As further discussed in Chapter Three, some parents become sexually interested in their youngsters when their bodies mature, whereas some parents and out-of-family molesters may find younger children more desirable as targets of sexual abuse (Quinsey, Rice, Harris, & Reid, 1993).

COMMON REACTIONS
TO ADOLESCENT ABUSE

Many abused adolescents present with a range of emotional and behavioral problems that might be addressed by the juvenile justice system, alternative services programs for runaway youths, or mental health departments. They may run away, steal, fail or skip school, fight, set fires, abuse drugs, or behave in other ways that cause them to be identified for services. Often these youths do not report themselves as in need of help, and are not identified by professionals, who perceive them as less vulnerable than younger children because of their age and size.

Many professionals do not view adolescent abuse as a significant problem. Child protective services workers with large caseloads and heavy demands on their time must make determinations about risk and imminent danger. If two reports of child abuse are phoned in at the same time, and the callers document concern regarding a toddler and an adolescent, chances are that the worker will appropriately prioritize the toddler for immediate response. Adolescents often have more resources than younger children, and may be able to get themselves to an emergency room for medical attention, seek shelter at a runaway facility, walk into a juvenile probation office, or seek help from others (extended family members, teachers, or family friends). Toddlers are unable to mobilize themselves in this manner and therefore require the immediate attention and protection of protective services workers. And yet when adolescents run away, or leave their families in the midst of crisis and conflict, they often resort to illegal means of self-care – prostitution, drug dealing, or other criminal activities. Often these youngsters find gang activity to provide valuable components of family life and feel accepted and cared for within gangs, regardless of whether the gang is or is not engaged in criminal activity.

In over 20 years of working in the area of child abuse prevention and treatment, I have had occasion to interact with many professionals and discuss their views about the work they do. Regarding child sexual abuse, I have heard professional comments that demonstrate differential responses to adolescent victims. For example, I heard one professional say, "That girl knew what she wanted and knew how to get it," in regard to a case of incest in which the father gave his daughter expensive gifts. In another case, in which the adult offender was female, I overheard an investigator call the adolescent victim "a lucky bastard" because he had had sexual intercourse with the 35-year-old mother of one of his friends.

I have also seen personal biases dictate responses. For example, two 16-year-olds engaged in heterosexual activity were seen as "healthy teens," whereas two 16-year-olds engaged in homosexual activity were referred to child protective services. Moreover, when adolescents are physically abused, varying responses occur as well. For example, a child with a black eye was once asked, "What did you do to bring that on?" Another adolescent girl was told that she had to "mind her parents better and not make them get so frustrated and angry."

Obviously, child neglect is most pertinent to young children who cannot meet their own needs. And yet adolescents may also suffer from parents who are inattentive and uninterested, and who choose to construct separate lives from their adolescents. One parent referred for counseling had set up a separate home for her 16-year-old because she did not want to share a home with the boy. She did not understand what the problem was, since the boy had been living "on his own" since he was about 10. Amazingly, the youngster had managed to get many of his needs met at school through positive relationships with his teachers. He excelled in school, and his pseudo-mature behavior projected an image of self-confidence and well-being that belied his feelings of loss, isolation, and longing.

Psychological abuse is probably one of the most common forms of child abuse, and yet only a handful of states consider it significant enough for intervention. There has been considerable controversy about how to define this particular form of abuse and how to intervene. However, several researchers suggest that psychological abuse, unaccompanied by physical or sexual abuse or neglect, also contributes to many long-term emotional and behavioral problems (Garbarino, Guttman, & Seeley, 1986).

In addition to varied professional responses at the intake level, legally mandated professionals may fail to report cases of adolescent abuse, so many situations go undetected and unreported. They may hesitate to report because they believe intervention will be minimal, or they have had past experiences in which their cases were not accepted. Also, they may be concerned about betraying adolescents' confidence, or they may fear incurring the wrath of angry youngsters or their irate parents.

We are left, therefore, with a significant problem that is often ignored or minimized, as well as a system whose interventions occur sporadically and appear cursory at best. At the same time, the long-lasting effects of childhood abuse continue to be documented as serious and far-reaching (Briere, 1989).

THE EFFECTS OF CHILDHOOD ABUSE ON ADOLESCENTS

Bagley (1995) states that

> prolonged and intrusive sexual abuse imposed on the physically immature body and the developmentally immature psyche of a child frequently creates an adolescent who cannot find adequate solutions to the dilemmas of identity development. . . . As a result, the adolescent is extremely vulnerable to stress, and may develop in severe form a number of the psychological disorders (e.g., suicidal ideas and behavior, depression, eating disorders, alienation from school and peers, sexual problems, acting-out behaviors, and substance abuse) that have an increasing prevalence among adolescents. . . . (p. 135)

Finkelhor and Dziuba-Leatherman (1994) cite the growing literature indicating that victimization has short- and long-term effects on children's mental health; they point out that sexually victimized children appear to be at a nearly fourfold increased lifetime risk for psychiatric disorders, and a threefold risk for substance abuse. Kolko (1992) also demonstrates increased rates of mental health morbidity for physical abuse; Briere and Runtz (1993) for psychological maltreatment; and M. A. Straus (1994) for corporal punishment. The proposition that childhood victims are more likely to grow up to victimize others, Finkelhor and Dziuba-Leatherman (1994) state, is firmly established.

Kendall-Tackett, Williams, and Finkelhor (1993) reviewed over 40 methodologically sound research studies of sexually abused children, seeking to ascertain whether a "profile" of sexually abused children would emerge. They found no such profile or "child sexual abuse syndrome," but did find that several symptoms appeared consistently across studies. These included symptoms of posttraumatic stress disorder (PTSD), especially fear and anxiety; depression; and problem sexual behaviors. Friedrich et al. (1992) state that open sexual behavioral problems are the most consistently identified effect of child sexual abuse. Schetky (1990) notes that the research on long-term effects of sexual abuse has also found psychiatric hospitalization, substance abuse, self-abuse, somatization disorder, eroticization, learning difficulties, dissociative disorders, conversion reactions, running away, prostitution, revictimization (even at the hands of mental health professionals [Kluft, 1990]), and impaired interpersonal relationships.

McCann, Pearlman, Sakheim, and Abrahamson (1988) discussing childhood abuse, state that because individuals "hold certain beliefs and expectations (schemata) about the self and others, which both shape and are shaped by the experiences of the world" (p. 78), disruptions occur in the schemata concerning safety, trust, power, and esteem. These disruptions in turn cause symptoms such as chronic anxiety and fear, confusion, overcaution, inability to trust others, chronic passivity, a sense of futility, depression, profoundly negative self-esteem, and feelings of guilt and shame.

Cuffe and Frick-Helms (1995) group the psychological issues involved in treating abused children into five cluster areas: guilt; betrayal; pseudomaturity and boundary confusion; self-mastery; and fear and other symptoms of PTSD. They note that 30–50% of sexually abused children can be diagnosed with PTSD, which is characterized by high levels of fear and anxiety, recurrent or intrusive memories, behavioral reenactments in play or behavior, emotional detachment and numbing, and an acute startle response.

Friedrich (1995a) finds that the impact of trauma occurs in three primary dimensions: attachment, self-regulation, and self-perspective. Attachment problems cause interactional problems in which children are often hesitant, emotionally distant or detached, and distrustful and hypervigilant. Self-regulation problems contribute to behavioral problems, such as violence, impulsivity, and sexual acting out, and explain the "lability and variability in the presentation of the sexually abused child" (p. 4). Lastly, Friedrich (1995a) states, "Self-perspective takes into consideration the child's developing sense of self and how aspects of the abuse experience are integrated into this sense of self and become part of one's self-representation" (p. 4). Putnam (1990) finds many disturbances of the self in abused children, including negative self-image, underdeveloped sense of identity, self-deprecation, a belief that they deserve the abuse, body image disturbances, self-destructive behavior, fragmentation, and concerns about control.

Friedrich (1995a) and Schetky (1990) note neurophysiological effects – for example, depletion of catecholamines, which they postulate results in psychological constriction and numbing, followed by a period of hyperarousal. These individuals may have a greater tendency to reexperience the initial trauma in the form of flashbacks or nightmares. Schetky (1990) suggests that the numbing and constriction that often follow trauma may also have a physiological base. Friedrich (1995a) notes that although the neurophysiological response to trauma is difficult for clinicians to identify or quantify, some symptomatic behaviors may be related, including sleep disorders, PTSD, attention-deficit/hyperactivity disorder, emotional lability/reactivity, compulsive behaviors, oppositionality, and dissociation. These symptoms have been documented in many studies of child sexual abuse victims (e.g., Waterman & Ben-Meir, 1993), as well as victims of other types of child abuse (Hart & Brassard, 1987; Wolfe, 1987; Jaffe, Wolfe, & Wilson, 1990).

It is important to note that child abuse does not appear to affect each victim in a predictable or consistent fashion (Cicchetti & Rizley, 1981). Certain variables may ameliorate or exacerbate the effects of the abuse. These include the duration of the abuse, relationship to the offender, affective content, type of sexual abuse, sex of the victim, age of the victim, age difference between victim and offender, sex of the offender, parental variables, and treatment (Schetky, 1990). Schetky summarizes:

> Long-lasting negative effects of childhood sexual abuse appear to be correlated with abuse by a father or a stepfather, use of force, and being unsupported by a close adult. It is highly probably that sexual activity that is intrusive and of long duration is most disruptive. School-age children seem to be at greatest risk for developing behavioral problems related to the abuse, at least in short-term studies. Girls are more likely than boys to show acute distress following sexual abuse, but data are lacking on which to make adequate comparisons between male and female victims in terms of long-term effects and adjustments. . . . Family support remains a critical variable with regard to outcome. (1990, pp. 40–41)

Although the most extensive research to date has been done on sexually abused children, Wolfe (1987), focusing on physically abused children, also finds them to have a greater than average risk of developing emotional and/or behavioral problems – particularly because of the disruption in the children's critical areas of development, such as attachment, self-control, and moral and social judgment. Wolfe further notes that physically abused children have problems in specific dimensions: the behavioral dimension (problems of self-control and aggression), the socioemotional dimension (deficits in social sensitivity and relationship development), and the social-cognitive dimension (issues in cognitive and moral development).

MITIGATING VARIABLES AND RESILIENCY

At the beginning of this chapter, I have chronicled the history of Jennifer, a 13-year-old single mother who had undergone physical abuse, sexual abuse, neglect, and emotional abuse. Remarkably, she was able to form a positive attachment to a foster mother, whose relationship with her extended beyond the formal foster parenting agreement.

From a review of Jennifer's history, it is difficult to fathom how and why she was able to cope and develop as well as she did. But the variable that struck me the most was her ability and willingness to trust. She had significant losses early on – she had felt great sadness at the loss of her biological mother, and the subsequent attachment she formed to her would-be adoptive mother, whom she also lost abruptly. Although she then made some efforts to detach herself from caretaking figures, she was responsive to positive attention and seemed to thrive as others talked with her and listened to her. Her ability to trust others after such acute violations of trust speaks volumes about her survival instinct. I believe that the presence of a significant other who provides consistency of empathic care and continuity of attention is one of the most important variables in mitigating the negative effects of childhood abuse, particularly because children seem to await positive interactions with great patience, and are often quite receptive to genuine concern.

Several times I have been impressed with how adolescents describe a teacher, a physician, a friend's parent, or some other adult who took the time to ask after them or converse, or who found their company worthwhile. Some youngsters greatly value the experience of someone's reaching out to them, being available to them, or sticking by them no matter what. This gives clinicians some important guidelines for maximizing the effectiveness of therapeutic contact.

Sanford (1990), in her well-titled book *Strong at the Broken Places,* describes the commonalities of many of the child and adult survivors of childhood abuse she has worked with:

> Despite popular and professional expectations, these survivors have not inflicted trauma on themselves or others. Their thoughts and feelings about childhood trauma are normal, given the abnormality of their experience. Their problems are not radically different in scope or intensity from those of many others I have worked with who were not traumatized as children. They leave therapy having resolved the issues that brought them and continue to live useful and rewarding lives. (p. xiv)

Motivated by her observations that some adult survivors fare better than others, she conducted a nonempirical and descriptive study of 20 healthy adults, each of whom extensively experienced at least two types of trauma (including physical and sexual abuse, parental substance abuse, extreme neglect, and the witnessing of domestic violence). Many of the adult survivors she interviewed found satisfaction and a sense of well-being in turning to work for a sense of identity and fulfillment – in doing so, they developed economic freedom, made social contacts, became productive and creative, and found jobs in which they could become helpful to others. In addition, they found and maintained their spirituality; they found strength in self-help programs; and they transformed their experiences into a greater appreciation of life, compassion for themselves, and caring for others.

Since some children seem to fare better than others, it is useful to consider mitigating variables. Waterman and Kelly (1993) studied what factors lessened the negative effects of trauma in 82 children, and conducted a 5-year follow-up of 40 of the original 82. They found that the following factors combined to promote healing: (1) a warm, supportive, nonpunitive, child-centered family; (2) less family tension and fewer stressors; (3) coping through mobilizing and reframing to increase family power; (4) close but not enmeshed families; and (5) decreased overt conflict and anger during problem solving.

Clearly, as clinicians, we are poised to provide valuable assistance to adolescents who can avail themselves of reparative and corrective experiences that might alter widespread negative beliefs about who they are, what the world has to offer, what interpersonal contacts can be like, how much personal power they have, and what they can or cannot change. In order to be helpful to adolescents with histories of current or past abuse, we must recognize the disruption in their developmental dimensions, the impact of trauma on them, and the nature and type of their psychological defenses. In addition, we must be aware of their resiliency issues and coping strategies, and constantly decode problem behavior in a way that is helpful to these youngsters.

THE PURPOSE OF THIS BOOK

The growing research on the impact of child abuse will continue to inform us regarding the type and extent of long-term consequences for victims of different ages and both genders, and for victims of different forms of abuse. Clinical observation will provide us with complementary data on common presenting problems and symptoms. And as we continue the dynamic process of learning about the population of abused adolescents, we must make efforts to deepen our understanding, formulate educated hypotheses about how to be helpful, incorporate research components that evaluate our clinical work (Finkelhor & Berliner, 1995), and exchange thoughts and ideas with our colleagues about how to mitigate the pervasive negative effects of childhood abuse.

The purpose of this book is to highlight the problems and concerns of adolescents who are currently abused, or who have histories of past abuse. My approach is to combine the information provided in the literature with my clinical experience to create, examine, refine, and implement useful strategies, grounded in a theoretical framework that includes material from developmental, attachment, systemic, and trauma theories. In particular, I believe that those adolescents' current behaviors, which may be identified as provocative or symptomatic, must be understood in the context of their past or current abuse. The basic premise is that child abuse interrupts and disrupts the developmental process, and that several developmental tasks are not fully addressed; therefore, these must be revisited during the treatment process.

In addition, I believe that *given certain discrete circumstances,* it is necessary to focus the therapy on past traumatic experiences that continue unresolved, and to do so for a specific period of time and in a structured manner. I propose a model of treatment that is primarily empowerment-based with a goal of increasing overall functioning, and is informed by therapy with adult survivors, particularly as proposed by Briere (1989, 1992), Courtois (1988), myself (Gil, 1988), and Herman (1992).

CHAPTER TWO

Theories of Adolescent Development

with Karren Campbell

A thorough knowledge of theories of development is essential for those who work with adolescents, particularly when it is likely that the developmental process of many such adolescents has been disrupted or compromised by maltreatment. A developmental framework is of great importance in assessing both the risk and the impact of victimization.

Finkelhor (1995) proposes that the types of victimization children suffer "depend on their age and level of development in a very basic way," and suggests that "how children respond to victimization depends on stage-specific capacities and vulnerabilities" (p. 178). He further states that risk may vary across the course of development, based on "1) the characteristics of children themselves [i.e., their suitability as targets and ability to protect themselves] and 2) the characteristics of environments they inhabit [i.e., the presence of people who want to victimize and the presence of capable guardians]" (p. 179). According to Finkelhor (1995), the impact of victimization can be affected by the child's stage of development in each of the following ways: "1) . . . as a result of the developmental tasks or developmentally critical periods the child is facing at the time of victimization, 2) . . . as a result of developmentally specific cognitive abilities of children that affect their appraisal of victimization, 3) . . . as a result of differences in the forms of symptom expression available to the child at particular stages of development" (p. 185). Thus, the effects of victimization can vary at different stages of development.

The relationship between risk and impact is complex, however. For example, let us consider the issue of self-protection. Wauchope and Straus (1990) found that only a third of 15- to 17-year-olds are hit by their parents, compared to 97% of 3-year-olds. They found that older children can often argue, placate, run away, or in some other way use size and age to equalize their position. However, in cases of chronic physical or sexual abuse, neglect, or emotional abuse, many youngsters' ability to protect themselves is compromised by what they perceive as "learned helplessness," or the futility of trying to stop long-standing abusive patterns. Victimization itself therefore may make some children more vulnerable and less able to experience personal control, options, or external resources, because it diminishes their self-esteem and sense of entitlement. If abuse is experienced during childhood (and carried forward into adolescence), several developmental tasks or processes are likely to have been compromised.

Although research on specific symptomatology of abuse by developmental age has just begun (Kendall-Tackett et al., 1993; Trickett & Putnam, 1993), abused adolescents appear to have a constellation of common symptoms, including depression, self-injurious behavior, running away, and substance abuse (Finkelhor, 1995).

Finkelhor concludes his important discourse on developmental victimology thus: "The need for new theory and research is vast and urgent, and ranges from how children view victimization at different ages and how it affects them, to what can be done to minimize their risk" (1995, p. 189).

AN OVERVIEW OF NORMAL ADOLESCENT DEVELOPMENT

Despite the relative dearth of theory and research in this area, the onus is on clinicians to apply their (imperfect) knowledge to their adolescent clients in light of each client's individual situation, and history. Even without a perfect theory, the existing information provides useful guidelines for assessment (Forehand & Wierson, 1993). All practitioners working with adolescents should have a thorough knowledge of normal development – that is, of the basic needs of children and adolescents, and the fundamental tasks confronting them at each stage of development.

A debate exists among researchers as to what normal adolescent development entails (M. A. Straus, 1994). Forehand and Wierson (1993) have pointed out that although none of the several existing theories are based on longitudinal studies of children's first 20 years of life, even if we had one unified theory based on such research, it could not pinpoint the precise transitions at specific ages. Given the abundance of racial, cultural, spiritual, regional, and other individual differences existing among cultures around the world and even within U.S. culture, this is not surprising.

Development is characterized by both continuous (the accumulation of behaviors and experiences over time) and discontinuous (age-specific plateaus and leaps in new skills) growth in physical, intellectual, and social dimensions (Janus et al., 1987). Major changes occur during adolescence, as evidenced by the difference between 12- or 13-year-olds in junior high school who are just reaching puberty, and 18-year-olds who may be steadily employed or have children (Barker, 1990).

Adolescence replicates and incorporates previously mastered stages of development, and may even be considered the final stage of childhood. Adolescents have rapid physical growth, as do infants; they expand their social horizons and develop their personalities, as do preschoolers; and they decrease family involvement while increasing peer and community involvement, as do youngsters in middle childhood (Weiner & Elkind, 1972). However, they also begin to explore different options in lifestyles, and the way in which others perceive them changes as they lose their status as children and begin to take on the characteristics of adulthood.

These rapid changes include affective development as well (Mann, Harmoni, & Power, 1989). It is normal for adolescents to fear a loss of control over their bodies, themselves, and their environments, and these fears are exaggerated by their mood changes and hormonal fluctuations (Singer, Singer, & Anglin, 1993). It should be noted, however, that the negative affect of adolescence is a less intense and more transitory mood state than the negative affect of clinical depression (Flannery et al., 1994).

Teenagers have to go beyond physical maturity if they are truly to become adults. This is done by gaining independence from their families, feeling secure in their sexual maturity, and establishing satisfactory and cooperative relationships with their peers. They must also select a meaningful vocation and prepare for it adequately (Congar, 1973, as cited in Janus et al., 1987).

In order to accomplish these tasks, adolescents need to achieve a sense of competence and autonomy. Many adolescent behaviors, such as questioning authority, are means through which adolescents learn to create their own interpretations and solutions to problems, rather than simply accepting adult explanations as before. Having flexible coping strategies and being able to behave appropriately in different situations are typical of healthy development.

The family is the primary environment in which an adolescent negotiates these tasks. Parents must gradually prepare for a healthy separation from their adolescent children. In Western society, the process of successful adolescent separation and development toward a responsible and enjoyable adulthood involves the whole family. Parents must change their methods of control, their attitudes, and their way of relating to encourage autonomy, or "the second individuation" (Blos, 1967). The goal is to establish involvement and encourage independence without being detached on the one hand, or smothering or rigid on the other.

Mixed feelings accompany the process of individuation for both parents and adolescents. Parents may be proud of their children's increasing physical, social, and intellectual achievements. At the same time, adolescents are vulnerable to failure and its inherent consequences, having rejected much of the parental protection that they received in childhood. For their part, parents must learn to overcome their frustrations sufficiently to allow their children the freedom to explore various areas as they learn to live their own lives. Economic, marital, health, social, and career difficulties, and the parents' own adolescent socialization, also affect the parent–child relationship (M. A. Straus, 1994). Discomfort, anxiety, guilt, and anger are typically felt by parents who have a hard time handling their children (Zarb, 1992).

Adolescents generally will take as much independence as they can get. Negotiations must be made among what parents will allow, what is good for the family, and what teenagers can handle (Corder, 1994). Healthy adolescents develop trust through having clearly defined expectations, although they may test these limits in order to establish how committed or concerned adults are (Merchant, 1990). Optimally, parents will be able to provide continued support, respecting their youngsters' ability, yet ready to help when the adolescents are unsure of how to handle a situation. The compromise between parents and adolescents may be in the form of bargaining, with rewards or punishment for a given behavior, mutual agreement on a set of rules, or unspoken demands or contracts.

Recommendations in the past that suggested early emotional detachment from one's family and less parental supervision are now recognized as inaccurate. Early separation actually provokes risk-taking behaviors with one's peers and antisocial activities. Premature distancing from parents can be caused by factors such as "early puberty, either authoritarian or permissive parenting, family disruption, large impersonal schools, and the availability of a negative peer culture" (Irwin, 1987, as cited in Hill, 1993, p. 71).

Among the results of an increasingly complex and technological world are more changes in family structure, such as divorce and/or remarriage, or adolescents' simply spending less time with their families. Although both children and adolescents are flexible in terms of such changes, stable, predictable environments are preferred (M. A. Straus, 1994). Adolescents who are less supervised are more vulnerable to negative outcomes such as violence. The burden of preparing adolescents for life and the job market has been unrealistically placed on the schools. Unemployed adolescents may be feared and derided because of the myth that industriousness is a moral quality.

Despite the realities of modern life and the fact that there may be no jobs for those who want them, such myths still prevail (M. A. Straus, 1994).

Also crucial is developing a philosophy of life over the course of adolescence – that is, a world view, moral standards, and guiding beliefs. "A basic philosophy is essential in lending order and consistency to the many decisions the individual will have to take in a changing, seemingly chaotic world. Before the adolescent can successfully abandon the security of childhood dependence on others, he must have some idea of who he is, where he is going and what the possibilities are of getting there" (Congar, 1973, p. 174, as cited in Janus et al., 1987, p. 21).

In sum, normal adolescent development, which follows its own progressive pattern (preadolescence, early adolescence, adolescence proper, and late adolescence) as described by Blos (1963), is characterized by healthy, productive growth and by development of the ability to plan an effective future. The eventual result is an adult who is a contributing member of society (Janus et al., 1987).

THEORIES ABOUT DIFFERENT
DIMENSIONS OF DEVELOPMENT

Crain (1992) provides a comprehensive analysis of the field of developmental psychology and has reviewed and summarized information on traditional developmental theories.

Developmental psychologists attribute the reason for the lack of one comprehensive theory to constant changes within economic, social, and cultural norms. For example, in medieval times children were seen as fully formed, miniature adults; they were treated like adults, and entered adult society by the age of 6 or 7. This was partly because egocentric adults assumed that everything had the same form and function as their own. Ariès (1960/1962), has also suggested that people may have been hesitant to cherish the unique qualities of children because of the high child mortality rates.

The 18th-century philosopher Jean Jacques Rousseau is considered the father of developmental psychology and introduced the idea of developmental stages, which is now common in most theories of development. What follows is a brief description of the major theories concerning different aspects of development.

Attachment

Because abused children by definition have negative parent–child interactions that might disrupt or interfere with the formation and positive function of attachment, developmental theory concerning attachment is of particular relevance. As a matter of fact, there is growing interest in attachment theory on the part of professionals specializing in the treatment of child abuse (James, 1995; Pearce & Pezzot-Pearce, 1994; Friedrich, 1995b).

John Bowlby (1969, 1973) stressed the importance of the mother–infant bond as a way to understand human development. He believed that if children are not given opportunities to form secure attachment to their mother figures early in life, the ensuing emotional problems may result in a lasting inability to form intimate, enduring relationships. Bowlby proposed that attachment behaviors, such as the gestures and signals that babies use (smiling, babbling, sucking, crying, grasping, and following), are environmentally adaptive for humans because they keep them close to their parents. As children grow, they develop secure attachments when they know that their parental figures are available, responsive, and willing to help in difficult situations (Barker, 1990). Such individuals feel bold and competent in their explorations of the world. So, according to Bowlby's theory, the need to have close attachments is built into human nature and allows future intimate ties with other people.

Mary Ainsworth and her colleagues (Ainsworth, Blehar, Waters, & Wall, 1978) extended Bowlby's attachment theory to ordinary child-rearing situations, making the application of the attachment theory to developmental tasks a bit easier. Ainsworth et al. hypothesized that infants can develop one normal attachment type (secure) or one of two abnormal attachment types (insecure/ambivalent and insecure/avoidant) with their mothers. These different attachment types are said to be predictive of later behavior. Securely attached children are persistent and curious in their play, whereas avoidant and ambivalent types exhibit various kinds of emotional difficulties.

"Internal working models" of attachment are important to attachment researchers. For example, Bowlby proposed that the internal working model consists of the child's expectations and feelings about the attachment figure's availability and responsiveness. But since internal working models involve thoughts and feelings, they are harder to study in infants. However, after about 3 years of age, infants can complete stories on attachment situations (e.g., a child's scraping his or her knee in a fall). Securely attached children tend to depict their parents as responsive and helpful; they are also not afraid to venture away from their parents and explore on their own. They are able to meet life with the greatest confidence when they know that there is a home base provided by their family or companions to which they can return. As Bowlby (1988) so aptly stated, individuals are at their happiest "when life is organized as a series of excursions, long or short, from a secure base provided by our attachment figures" (Bowlby, 1988, p. 62).

Adolescents and adults who are attached in an avoidant or ambivalent manner typically have emotional difficulties, as noted above. Avoidant individuals may have problems developing close relationships, whereas ambivalent individuals may be overly dependent and depression-prone.

Karen (1994) remains guardedly optimistic about working with adolescents regarding attachment problems. He states,

> One way or another, it would seem important to reach insecurely attached children by adolescence, because that's when it is believed their patterns become more firmly set. Even then they can still be changed; there is still the possibility of psychotherapy, not to mention other vital relationships, and the emotional flux of the adolescent years sometimes opens children up in new ways. (p. 232)

Cognitive Development

Cognitive distortions permeate the adult abuse survivor's thinking. They shape his or her beliefs about why the abuse occurred; how it might have been prevented; what it means about the individual's lovability, worthiness, and ability to control his or her environment; and what can be expected from the future.

Some research suggests that adolescents may be better able to cope with sexual abuse than younger children may be. Gomes-Schwartz, Horowitz, and Sauzier (1985) found that incestuous experiences with onset during teenage years were more likely to involve some degree of consent, and teens were better able to process the experience intellectually. On the other hand, cognitive processes may be interrupted by distressing or traumatic experiences, and will be affected by abuse experiences that occur much earlier in childhood. In my experience, we greatly overestimate adolescents' cognitive abilities where child abuse is concerned, because they are generally compromised by dependency on, and love for, those who maltreat them. I believe that some abused adolescents do not receive proper intervention as a result of an exaggerated reliance on their cognitive abilities to assess child abuse properly.

Assumptions about cognitive ability at different life stages are based on theories of "normal" cognitive development. Piaget's cognitive-developmental theory is the most thorough and integrated theory proposed in this area thus far (Piaget, 1970, 1971, 1972). He divided development into four general periods: (1) sensorimotor intelligence (birth to 2 years); (2) preoperational thought (2 to 7 years); (3) concrete operations (7 to 11 years); and (4) formal operations (11 years to adulthood). Children pass through these periods at different rates and ages, but certain increasingly comprehensive methods of thinking occur in the same order. Piaget did not believe that these changes are genetically predetermined or that thinking is influenced by environmental factors or teaching; rather, he believed that cognitive changes are most influenced by children themselves. He proposed that although interaction with the environment is a requisite for development, children's own activities control the bulk of their cognitive development as their abilities naturally become more and more differentiated and complex.

It is not until individuals attain formal operations that thinking may be completely abstract or hypothetical. Piaget posited that because adolescents can think about more comprehensive problems, their social lives are characterized by more thought about their futures and social integration. These thoughts lead to utopian and idealistic thinking, including abstract principles such as love, liberty, and justice.

Adolescents thus begin to imagine and dream of hypothetical situations and societies, constructing perfect worlds. This idealistic thinking is related to what Piaget called a different type of egocentrism than that seen in infants and children – one that develops because of the broad spectrum of possibilities generated by adolescents' thought processes. Without testing their thoughts in reality, teenagers may believe that their thoughts have unlimited power and that they can transform their futures or the world through their ideas. Piaget believed that adolescents can only lose their egocentrism, or become "decentered," when they adopt adult roles that teach them the limitations on their thoughts; only then will they be able to see that the value of such thoughts depends on how things operate in reality. This egocentrism may contribute to risky behaviors in adolescents, who often seem to believe that dangerous behaviors will not result in catastrophes, or will affect others and not themselves. It may also be this egocentrism that causes adolescents to disregard the impact of current experiences or behaviors. A national 1992 household survey of 10,645 youths from 12 to 21 released by the National Center for Health Statistics (1995) indicates that adolescents engage in a broad range of risky behaviors, including unprotected sex, tobacco and alcohol use, and driving while intoxicated, among other things.

Piaget believed that changes in cognitive ability lend themselves to the identity searching and self-questioning often seen in adolescence. Adolescents may think about limitless options in terms of who they are now and who they will be. However, formal operational thinking is not characteristic of all adolescent thinking, and may be used only in situations in which a young person is most interested. (Even adults do not regularly exhibit this type of thinking unless they too are interested in a particular area.) In adolescence, the focus of moral decision making also shifts from consequences to intentions. Whereas a younger child might base a decision about right and wrong on the amount of damage a person has done in a situation (i.e., greater damage is assigned more severe consequences), the older child looks at the person's underlying motive and intentions to determine how wrong that individual is (Crain, 1992). Adolescents consider more possibilities in problem solving, thinking with logic and flexibility. To do this, however, they require models and compelling situations for different ways to solve problems (M. A. Straus, 1994).

Newton (1995) discusses changes that occur in the brain during adolescence, including "discrete changes at cell synapse and morphological levels," and the "associational or system level" changes that cause a series of important systemic changes in the brain (p. 33). As mentioned in Chapter One, findings of recent research on sexually abused children also reveal changes in brain functioning as a result of the demands of external stressors; these may unsettle or delay brain development in adolescence.

Moral Development

Moral development is endangered by children's experience of abuse and neglect, because issues of justice, right and wrong, and fairness are clearly compromised. Abused children learn the discrepancies between those who have power and those who do not, and they often identify with the role of the aggressor, which may be viewed as more rewarding. When children are raised in environments characterized by inconsistency, chaos, lack of boundaries, inattention, and/or blunt force, their ideas about morality are bound to be affected.

Lawrence Kohlberg (1981) proposed that children develop increasingly complex methods for exploring and trying to understand their environments. He proposed six stages of moral development, over the course of which individuals shift from unhesitating obedience of authority to concern with motives and the relative nature of moral dilemmas.

At the preconventional level (first two stages), individuals see morality as something external that is imposed upon them. In the first stage of moral development, children obey powerful authority figures without question. In the second stage, they can differentiate between right and wrong; however, they act mainly to avoid punishment (external control), rather than on the basis of an internalized sense of right and wrong.

Children entering their teens are capable of conventional morality, the second level (third and fourth stages) of moral thinking. Youngsters in the third stage are more aware of the needs of others; in the fourth stage, they are also able to consider the needs of society as a whole, and to see why certain rules and laws are necessary to maintain order.

People reaching the postconventional level (fifth and sixth stages) are capable of the most highly developed moral thinking. In the fifth stage, individuals are able to differentiate between social rules and laws on the one hand, and basic human rights and values that are more important than social laws on the other. Finally, those people who attain the sixth and last stage of moral development are aware of universal principles of morality, and are capable of understanding the relative nature of justice (e.g., the fact that democratic principles are not always fair to all members of society).

Like Piaget, Kohlberg stressed that these stages do not develop as a result of maturation, genetic predispositions, or socialization, and that there are no set ages at which an individual moves through the stages. Socialization by parents, teachers, and others arouse mental processes by challenging incomplete positions. Such challenges may cause the child to achieve a higher level of moral thinking, but moving through the stages is the result of the individual's thinking about moral dilemmas, not of socialization itself. The best development occurs when children are not forced to conform, but are allowed to resolve their own differences and to develop their own opinions. If they are not stimulated, however, individuals may not reach higher stages of reasoning. Once they do, they can understand and incorporate the understanding that they have gained from previous stages.

Kohlberg believed that these stages are universally applicable across all cultures, because, despite people's differing beliefs, their underlying methods of reasoning are the same. They may, however, pass through stages at differing rates, and terminate moral reasoning at different stages. In the United States, most urban, middle-class adults are said to use stage 4 reasoning, while few are thought to use stage 5 reasoning. Although there is some relationship between an individual's moral thoughts and actions, it is not clear how strong that relationship is or what causes it (Crain, 1992).

Closely linked to moral development is spiritual development, or adolescents' "quest for the meaning of life" (Newton, 1995, p. 86), in which they may question moral rules vis-à-vis a "higher power"; the existence and definition of a deity; a sense of ecology with larger humanity; and involvement with traditional, structured religious practices. Spirituality can be helpful in providing external controls as well as internal sources of strength and calm.

Physical Development

"Puberty" refers to the rapid physical changes and growth that occur in adolescence. Because of the progressively earlier onset of physical development in recent times, many adolescents seek sexual and financial independence earlier, even though they remain at least partially financially dependent on their parents for longer periods of time (often staying in school until young adulthood). It is important to recognize that although puberty is a part of one's sexual and reproductive development, it is not the beginning of sexuality (Peterson & Taylor, 1980). Sexuality is a normal process throughout childhood (Johnson, 1993) that takes a more central focus during adolescence. Some believe that being able to establish intimacy with another individual is the desired outcome of adolescent sexual development, rather than intercourse per se. However, since emotional, cognitive, and intellectual development are slower than physiological development, teens may become sexually active before they are ready to handle the consequences.

According to Bukowski, Sippola, and Brender (1993),

> The physical metamorphoses of puberty are among the most salient transitions of adolescence and can be a source of concern, anxiety, and preoccupation for many youngsters. Because these

concerns may be accentuated by the changing perceptions of others toward the adolescent, there may also be a transformation of the self-concept in response to the internal and external reactions to their changing physical appearance. Many of these responses reflect an increasing awareness, by the adolescent and by others, of the individual's sexuality. (p. 95)

As will be seen in Chapter Three, some cases of abuse are long-standing, with adolescents having been abused throughout their lives. However, other types of abuse are specifically related to this phase of development, some of which are precipitated by the overt physical signs of sexuality that emerge during this time. It is clear from the literature that sexual abuse has an undeniable impact on children's developing sexuality, although the extent and type of effects vary from child to child. Several studies of sexually abused children have found disturbances in sexual identity and sexual functioning (Browne & Finkelhor, 1986; Coons, 1986), promiscuity (Courtois, 1979), and disturbances in sexual orientation (Burgess, Hartman, & McCormack, 1987). Precocious sexual behaviors and eroticization are the most common signs of sexual abuse (Friedrich, Urquiza, & Beilke, 1986). Bukowski et al. (1993) state that "sexual development in adolescence consists of a constellation of phenomena that ultimately fits within an individual's personal matrix of experience and meaning" (p. 93). A thorough understanding of normative sexual development is required in order to gauge the differentiating behaviors provoked by early sexual abuse (Martinson, 1991; Bukowski et al., 1993; Culley & Flanagan, 1995).

Adolescents achieve approximately 25% of their adult height during the growth period of puberty, as well as about 40% of their optimum adult weight (Singer et al., 1993). Structural changes in both males and females include genital growth (i.e., an increase in the size of penis and testes, or lengthening of the vagina), as well as increased levels of certain hormones in the blood. Other physiological changes include the production of sperm in the testes for males, changes in the ovaries that lead to menses for females, changes in the pulmonary and circulatory systems, and the maturation of the hypothalamic–pituitary system (Bukowski et al., 1993).

The changes in puberty occur in a consistent pattern. In females, breast development occurs first, between the ages of 8 and 13 (at age 11 on the average), and is followed by the growth of pubic hair. After breast development and the growth spurt in height and weight are well under way, menarche (often considered the evidence of "womanhood") begins between the ages of 10 and 16.5, with a mean onset age of 12.8 years (Singer et al., 1993).

Physical changes in males start 1 or 2 years later than in females, beginning between 9.5 and 13.5 years of age, at an average age of 11.6. The first signs are an increase in the size of the testes and scrotum, and the growth of pubic hair. Increased height is accompanied by the enlargement of the penis and by darker, coarser pubic hair. Later in puberty, facial hair grows; the voice deepens because of growth of the larynx; and "nocturnal emissions" or "wet dreams" and the ability to ejaculate during masturbation occur (Bukowski et al., 1993). These last changes can be a source of concern for sexually naive males.

Both genders require approximately 3–5 years to complete the discomforting and rapid development of puberty. Puberty typically occurs earlier and is completed sooner in girls than in boys. Females complete their development of secondary sex characteristics within 1 to 2.5 years, while males may take 2 to 4.5 years. Of course, the pattern, timing, and rate of changes during puberty vary widely among individuals. Puberty can occur as early as age 10 and as late as age 17, but such extremes are unusual. Recent findings by Putnam and colleagues (Putnam, 1991) associate sexual abuse with precocious puberty. These findings coincide with my clinical experience. I have worked with very young children (5 and 7 years of age) who began their menses, as well as two girls who were pregnant by the age of 9. All these children had histories of severe and chronic sexual abuse.

Adolescents' self-confidence, body image, psychological development, and social development are affected by the wide individual differences in onset and rate of pubertal development, especially if they are different from what appears to be normal. There is a curvilinear relationship between pubertal development and body image in females (Tobin-Richards, Boxer, & Petersen, 1983). That is, compared to on-time and late maturers, early-maturing females (aged 11 to 12) have a negative body image, experience social difficulties (Chilman, 1983), and report the highest levels of sad affect (Flannery et al., 1994); late maturers also see their bodies more negatively than do those who mature on time, and social norms for appearance affect their self-image (Bukowski et al., 1993; Chilman, 1983).

Pubertal changes in females are not only uncomfortable, but have less favorable social value than such changes in males (Tobin-Richards et al., 1983). Menarche, the onset of menstrual periods (Singer et al., 1993), may cause some girls to feel "more womanly" (Koff, 1983), and to show more sexual differentiation of identity (Rierdan & Koff, 1980). Yet some girls may lose self-esteem and see boys as attaining more power at this time (Delaney, Lupton, & Toth, 1988). They may perceive a power differential because menarche is seen as a negative event in North American culture, and the girls themselves may see it as a "hygienic crisis" that appears at inconvenient times and restricts their activities. However, other changes during puberty may be viewed differently; for example, breast development is related to higher adjustment scores, as well as more positive body images and peer relationships.

Early development in boys may be a social advantage that can continue through their high school years. Boys who mature much earlier see their bodies more positively than those who are on time or late (Tobin-Richards et al., 1983). The onset of ejaculation, or spermache, may also be a positive experience, causing a boy to feel grown up, excited, happy, proud, curious, or surprised. Parents may also tolerate more independence (though they may discourage emotional displays), and may subtly encourage sexual activities when their sons develop (Tobin-Richards et al., 1983, as cited in Bukowski et al., 1993).

Although sexuality and its development begin at birth and extend through the lifespan, many people have their first interpersonal sexual experience in adolescence (Barbaree, Marshall, & Hudson, 1993), and romantic relationships are likely to begin developing in midadolescence (Zarb, 1992). Even when parents disapprove of early sexual experiences, adolescents determine their own moral values about responsible behavior in given situations. Their standards for handling sexual behavior may be different from those of their parents, which may cause conflict and hinder discussions about options for birth control, safe sex, or avoiding communicable diseases (Corder, 1994).

Of course, society also has expectations about adolescents' sexuality. The mass media tout a "pseudomature" image of their sexuality (e.g., a controversy emerged during the preparation of this book regarding suggestive Calvin Klein ads featuring what appeared to be preadolescent models), whereas adults may deny their sexuality altogether. Adults often tend to imagine, and be anxious about, the erotic and sexual behavior of adolescents.

Transitions in the way youngsters look, in the way they think, in the way they behave in social contexts, in their social and legal status, in their relationships with family and peers, in their achievements, in their feelings of identity, and in their independence and autonomy all characterize adolescence. Not surprisingly, sexual development in adolescence has an impact on nearly all of these areas. Sexuality is not just a physical or behavioral phenomenon; it is multidimensional and is part of identity formation.

To get used to their changing bodies, adolescents must learn their physical limitations and capabilities, understand their sexual/reproductive abilities, and integrate these into their interpersonal relationships (Janus et al., 1987). Males may express sexual behavior earlier than females, but both genders progress from sexual urges to feeling attracted to others, then dating, holding hands, fondling, and eventually intercourse (Schofield, 1965). This fairly predictable sequence may occur over 1–2 years. However, African-American teens may exhibit a shorter sequence, which may follow a different course (Smith, 1989). Individual differences may also be attributable to hormonal factors (i.e., levels of testosterone and estrogen); social factors such as peers' sexuality; and the degree of commitment in a relationship, which increases the acceptable range of sexual experience (Smith, Udry, & Morris, 1985). Of course, the likelihood of an adolescent's being sexually active is influenced not only by his or her level of physical maturation and the sexual maturity of peers, but also by how sexually attractive the adolescent is.

Thus the social, physical, psychological, and behavioral aspects of sexuality must be integrated with prior experiences, expectations, subjective meanings, emotions, and personal motives (Gagnon, 1972). Many different factors must be taken into account in this process of integration: "feelings of sexual desire and interpersonal attraction, one's sense of morality, social convention, interpersonal security, and one's view of others as sexual beings who have their own needs, desires and rights" (Bukowski et al., 1993, p. 86). Adolescents who have been sexually abused and exploited must also integrate a healthy respect for their own needs, desires, and rights, particularly the right to accept or reject others' sexual attention.

Sexual feelings and relationships may lead adolescents to feel confused and anxious. They may desire to be involved in relationships, but may be shy and lack confidence. They commonly fear sexual inadequacy or rejection. Conversely, some adolescents may become sexually active early in an attempt to fill their need for love, security, and affiliation (Barker, 1990).

According to Weiner and Elkind (1972), teenagers are confronted with three types of conflicts involving sexuality, intimacy, and security. The sexuality versus security conflict involves safely handling sexual urges—satisfying both their need to explore their sexuality and their need for emotional security. In the intimacy versus sexuality conflict, they learn to safely become friends with individuals to whom they are sexually attractive. Then, in the intimacy versus security conflict, they need to find intimacy outside (and inside) of their families without being hurt.

Similarly, Bukowski et al. (1993) proposed six requirements for developing a healthy sense of sexuality: learning about intimacy from one's peers; understanding personal roles and relationships in and out of the home; adjusting one's body schema or understanding as one's physical size, shape, and capabilities change; adjusting to and incorporating erotic feelings and experiences; learning social practices and standards of sexual expression; and understanding and appreciating the reproductive process.

Psychosexual Development: Freud's Theory

Unlike other formal theories of development (which deal with physical, motor, or other aspects of development), Sigmund Freud's psychoanalytic theory (Freud, 1935, 1954) attempts to explain impulses, fantasies, and feelings. Freud proposed that psychological change (and thus development) is controlled by internal forces such as biological maturation. Social factors are also important in his theory, in that he felt that sexual and aggressive forces caused by biological maturation need to be adapted for use in society. His theory about psychosexual development continues to be widely used even today as a basis for understanding of sexual development.

Sexual feelings, which are any feelings that create bodily pleasure, are very active in early childhood, yet are diffuse and very general. Though nearly any part of one's body can become the site on which sexual energy is focused, the mouth, the anus, and the genital area are the three most important zones in childhood sexuality. Each area represents a specific stage of sexual development and interests for the child. The oral and anal stages occur first, but according to Freud, it is the third stage – the phallic or Oedipal stage – that is pivotal in the formation of sexual identity. This stage occurs between the ages of 3 and 6 years. During this time, boys compare their penises to the penises of other males and animals; they may find pleasure in showing their penises to others; and they imagine themselves as adult males. A little boy's experiments and his fantasies of being a heroic and aggressive male are frequently directed at the mother, his primary love object. He may aggressively kiss her, desire to sleep in her bed at night, and have fantasies of marrying her, though he is probably unaware of sexual intercourse. He sees quickly that these plans and behaviors are not appropriate, and he resents his father, who does with his mother what he would like to do. The Oedipus complex (or competition with the father for the mother) is said to begin as a result of this conflict. The little boy then develops jealousy and fear of doing harm to his father, despite his love for this parent. He develops defensive maneuvers (such as burying his sexual feelings and verbalizing pure love for the mother, while repressing hostility for the father and trying to be more like him) in order to deal with his fear of being castrated for his behavior. Overcoming the Oedipal crisis is accomplished by internalizing a superego or conscience (i.e., adopting as his own the moral prohibitions of his parents, which cause guilt and serve to keep his behavior in check).

For girls, a form of the Oedipal complex is also said to occur (it is referred to as the Electra complex); however, Freud admitted that in this area, his theory is incomplete. He did note that by 5 years of age, girls become disappointed in their mothers and feel deprived because the constant love and attention they required as babies have decreased. Girls also become more irritated with their mothers' restrictions on their behaviors, including masturbation. Freud claimed that mothers are blamed by little girls for the girls' not having penises and thus being inadequately equipped from birth. A little girl recovers her feminine pride by beginning to enjoy the attention that her father gives her as a result of her developing femininity and cuteness; she develops romantic fantasies about her father, including an obscure wish for her father's penis and soon a desire to have a baby that she can give as a gift to her father.

Like the little boy, the little girl too realizes that she cannot marry, hug, cuddle, or sleep with her father as much as she would like to. Her mother becomes her competitor for the affections of her father when she realizes that her mother can do these things. However, whereas Freud believed that the motivation of castration fear leads to resolution for boys, the motivation for girls is unclear. Although Freud admitted to not knowing the answer, he guessed that it involves a fear of the loss of parental love, causing the girl to identify with her mother (by repressing desires), and to control her impulses and wishes by instituting her superego.

During latency age, the fourth stage of Freud's psychosexual theory, children aged 6 to 11 years, build strong defenses against Oedipal feelings. Both sexual and aggressive fantasies are suppressed in the unconscious, as well as oral and anal memories. Children are calm and unbothered because they have suppressed their dangerous impulses and are free to redirect their energy into sports, games, and intellectual activities that are socially acceptable. Though a child may be interested in the bodies of the gender to which he or she is attracted and may learn about the "facts of life," sexual concerns are not scary and overwhelming, and the child is able to maintain self-control and composure.

Puberty begins at approximately age 11 for girls (and at about age 13 for boys). At this time, during the fifth and final genital stage, adult-like sexual energy is experienced and threatens the established defenses of the adolescent. Not only are Oedipal feelings trying to break into consciousness, but the adolescent is now physically large enough to fulfill them; sexual interests are again focused on the genital region. Freud saw the largest responsibility of adolescents as getting free from their parents. However, this independence is not easily won because of the intense dependency on their parents that has developed through the years. Thus emotional separation is painful, and most people never attain complete independence.

Personality Development and Identity Formation

Of critical importance to adolescent development is the formation of a sense of self. It appears that individuals who are abused have impaired self-reference, including the absence of an internal base or model for behavior (Briere & Runtz, 1993). Westen (1994) also notes that abused children may shut down their capacity to think about their own thoughts and behaviors. Similarly, Linehan (1993) finds that abused children are often incapable of observing themselves accurately and may be prone to behave in ways that are incongruous and unpredictable. Cole and Putnam (1992) state that sexually abused children have problems with defining and integrating different aspects of the self, and as a result may have difficulties with social functioning, disturbances in body image, loss of memory about the self, and/or a sense of separate or fragmented selves.

The development of a sense of self is not an isolated process and depends on interaction from others. If others are critical, inconsistent, or harsh, children may feel invalidated. Benedict and Zantra (1993) found that the home environments of many sexually abused children add to their problems in self-formation. Adolescents are mostly concerned with not being acceptable to others and worrying about their place in society; Friedrich (1995b) notes that abused children and adolescents often feel a sense of *differentness*, shame over the abuse, and an assumption of responsibility for the abuse. Obviously, events that make children feel stigmatized will affect their self-images.

Since adolescents' mental abilities are also expanding, they may be able to imagine the many options available or not available to them, which in itself may be overwhelming. Early abuse may contribute to young persons' sense of futility about what they can and cannot accomplish; they often have a sense of decreased power and control (Friedrich, 1995b). Friedrich goes on to note that abused children and adolescents have specific symptoms reflecting self-related issues, including unstable sense of self, marked identity problems, multiple personality disorder, somatization disorder, distorted body image, reduced self-efficacy, atypical depression, and borderline features.

Again, the degree to which the self is compromised by abuse is most easily assessed in relation to current knowledge about normal development. Erikson's (1963) highly respected theory about the development of personality covers the development of identity and sense of self. His proposed eight stages of life incorporate information on socialization and cross-cultural development into a representation of global development during each stage.

According to Erikson, the first year of life is especially important for developing a sense of trust versus mistrust. A sense of trust emerges from a secure attachment to the parent. Over the next few years, children develop a sense of autonomy versus shame and a sense of initiative versus guilt when they are encouraged and supported by their parents in their exploration of the world around them. Children beginning school must negotiate the stage of industry versus inferiority; if they feel successful in their endeavors, they develop a sense of competence in their abilities to deal with the world. Adolescence is marked by the conflict between identity and role confusion. Once individuals have negotiated this stage, they are able to proceed to the next two stages of young adulthood and adulthood: intimacy versus isolation, and generativity versus self-absorption.

Erikson believed that the primary task for adolescents is to create a sense of ego identity – to come to know who they are and to work toward taking their place in society. Blos (1967) likewise emphasized the achievement of a workable self-acceptance, which includes an understanding and acceptance of inner complexities, as well as the ability to relate to others both interpersonally and in the context of a larger society.

Identity formation is a process that extends over a lifetime, but adolescence is the central point for its development, and various aspects of previous identities appear insufficient for the decisions that adolescents must now make. Positive and long-lasting ego identity (a sense of the self in the world as complete and separate; M. A. Straus, 1994) is also formed through accomplishments such as physical, academic, artistic, and other achievements that have cultural value. Adolescents must create "some central perspective and direction, some working unity, out of the effective remnants of [their] childhood and the hopes of [their] anticipated adulthood" (Erikson, 1958, p. 14, as cited in Crain, 1992, p. 257).

Erikson (1963) noted that though identity formation is mostly achieved through an unconscious process, teenagers frequently realize to their discomfort that they often cannot make lasting commitments and yet that they have many decisions to make that affect their futures. This difficulty may lead some into a psychosocial moratorium – a period during which they try to find themselves, take time off from school, try different jobs, or travel before they make important decisions about their futures. (Erikson failed to consider that economically disadvantaged youths do not have this luxury.) During this time, however, adolescents may feel isolated, worry that they are wasting time, feel that there is little meaning in what they are doing, or come to believe that they are not fully in control of their destinies.

Other adolescents accept defined social roles prematurely in an effort to establish some sense of self (identity foreclosure). Extended attempts to form identity may be painful, yet may result in higher levels of personal integration as well as true social strengths. Adolescents who struggle to find a lifestyle to which they can truly commit themselves, developing qualities such as loyalty or fidelity to people and beliefs, may eventually establish a more well-defined sense of identity.

Societal Demands and Social Development

In order to develop as individuals and to contribute to society, adolescents must be able to develop satisfying relationships with others shifting from an "egocentric to sociocentric orientation" (Newton, 1995, p. 124). In fact, making choices about the types of social groups to which one belongs is a natural part of life at all ages.

Social development is integrally linked to identity formation. Relationships with peers are a fundamental part of the development of a sense of competence and autonomy as adolescents become individuals in their own right, separate from their parents and families. Boundaries, or invisible lines, exist around all relationships within the family, defining who belongs within the family. Adolescents test these boundaries when they introduce their peers into their families and spend more time outside of their families (Singer et al., 1993).

Clearly, a large number of factors can affect a child's social development. Albert Bandura's social learning theory describes how children become functioning members of society (Bandura & Walters, 1963). Bandura emphasizes the role of social conditioning—that is, the ways in which parental child-rearing techniques, cultural and social expectations (of peers and family members), and certain models (parents, teachers, and increasingly peers and entertainment heroes) all exert a significant influence on children. In addition, Bandura and colleagues assert that aggression can be transmitted through imitative behavior with aggressive models (Bandura, Ross, & Ross, 1961). This has clear implications for youth who are abused or witness violence in the family.

Identifying with one's peer group is central to the development of self-esteem and social skills (Singer et al., 1993). Interpersonally, adolescents must come to understand what is needed to experience healthy intimacy with others, to be able to get close to people, to express their feelings, and to touch people of either gender (Corder,

1994). As orientation toward one's peers increases in early adolescence, the number of friends increases; peer conformity is highest for early adolescents (Hill, 1993).

Peer groups can range in size from a few to 20 or more members. Members may identify themselves as a group by developing and using slang expressions (Barker, 1990). These peer relationships are also crucial to developing the capacity for intimacy, as adolescents learn to "reveal the self" to one another (Singer et al., 1993). While developing interpersonal skills, adolescents appear to be more comfortable in same-sex groups when they are 13 years of age or younger; older adolescents seem to enjoy feedback from members of the opposite sex, but do not enjoy being the only person of their gender in a group (Corder, 1994).

Middle adolescents spend more time with their peers, especially outside of school (Hill, 1993). Peers become more central to teenagers' lives as the teenagers decrease their dependence on their parents and their families in general. Peers support one another through the challenges of this developmental period (Barker, 1990), and supply one another with most of their reinforcement and value systems (Hill, 1993). Though adolescents may lack self-confidence, peers may enable the adolescents to attempt things that they would not try on their own. Peers can influence socially responsible behavior, maturity, and healthy personality development (Barker, 1990).

Of course, peers may also have an equally harmful influence in many ways. Since many adolescents are referred to treatment when their behavior becomes a problem to others, it is important to view the problem behavior in the context of motivation. When adolescents identify with "in-groups," and become intolerant, cruel, and exclusionary to people different from themselves, they are attempting to find an identity by stereotyping themselves and what they believe at the moment. In particular, it seems that many adolescents seek membership in groups out of longing to belong to a larger system that values or cares for its members. They may also be motivated by political or religious theories: Through peer group activities, they search for values that they can uphold. However, peer groups can stifle individuality when they demand conformity from their members. If an individual is unable or unwilling to conform to such demands, the individual may experience anxiety, rejection from the group, and damaged self-esteem (Barker, 1990).

CONCLUSIONS

Despite the complexity and ambiguity of some of the issues discussed in this chapter, the good news is that adolescence offers wonderful opportunities (M. B. Straus, 1994) and can be an extremely joyful and exciting developmental stage. Adolescents struggling with disheartening pathogens have much to look forward to on their road to wellness. As M. B. Straus (1994) points out, adolescence, at its simplest, is just one of the various stages through which we pass on our journey from birth to old age. Of course, we would be naive to rely on this simplistic an explanation; however, given the complexity of the issues that adolescents must face, it may be far too easy "not to see the forest for the trees," and to become weighed down by hopelessness, frustration, and bureaucracy.

Two things are very clear: Adolescents face tremendous demands for growth in a variety of dimensions during this developmental phase, and they can be either helped or hindered by their families, environments, and experiences. Although adolescence does not have to be a difficult, overwhelming, and chaotic period of life, for too many adolescents it is a time fraught with family conflict, isolation, involvement in risky behaviors, and a general sense of "wandering."

As clinicians working with adolescents who are referred to treatment, we must evaluate their symptoms or problem behaviors, in a much larger context, which includes developmental, social, and family demands and obstacles. We will often be in positions of advocating for social changes that might create safer or more nurturing (supportive) environments for our young clients, or in other ways help these youngsters remove obstacles impeding their natural growth.

Adolescents are probably the most challenging and rewarding clients. They can alternate between being provocative and demanding on the one hand, and compliant and receptive on the other. Once positive therapeutic relationships are developed, adolescents are often capable of making constructive use of therapy very rapidly. They often simply need someone to believe in them and care for them in order to believe in themselves and take steps on their own behalf.

As a final note, it is predicted that in the United States, because of demographic shifts, approximately 30% of adolescents will be members of ethnic minority groups by the year 2000 (Hill, 1993). More socioeconomic, racial, and ethnic variables need to be studied in this area (M. B. Straus, 1994). However, most of the information available on adolescent development either summarily mention or ignore issues related to diversity in ethnicity, religious beliefs, sexuality, acculturation, and so forth. Although this book does not focus on this information, these factors must be kept in mind and explored in work with adolescent clients. Recent efforts to document culturally sensitive work with children and adolescents may signal future development of materials that broaden our understanding of cultural variables, and contribute to the enhancement of culturally sensitive therapeutic approaches (Vargas & Koss-Chioino, 1992).

CHAPTER THREE

Current versus Cumulative Abuse of Adolescents

As noted in Chapter One, there is ample evidence that abuse and neglect have the potential for more or less severe effects on a child's cognitive, behavioral, physical, emotional, psychological, neuropsychological, moral, and spiritual development. Child abuse compromises a youngster's sense of identity, safety, and personal power, and can create far-reaching consequences throughout development (Briere & Runtz, 1993). And although studies on the immediate and long-term consequences of abuse (particularly physical and sexual abuse) have been plentiful, there has been a paucity of research focusing specifically on abused adolescents; this may reflect the lack of concern about the plight of older youngsters, who are perceived by many as less vulnerable, more resourceful, and more capable of self-protection than younger children.

There are in fact two groups of abused adolescents: those who have been abused from childhood throughout many developmental stages, and those who are abused for the first time during their adolescent years—adolescents may be vulnerable to abuse because of their age, or due to family conflict or inconsistent child-rearing patterns. In this chapter, I discuss what I believe to be differential effects of current versus cumulative abuse on adolescents.

DISTINGUISHING CURRENT
FROM CUMULATIVE ABUSE

The abuse of adolescents either occurs in direct relationship to their developmental age and stage, or is a continuation of earlier patterns of child maltreatment. It is valuable to assess whether adolescent abuse is acute or chronic. Acute abuse may be precipitated by adolescent developmental issues (differentiation, autonomy, identity, and transition); these issues may provoke parental fear, confusion, or volatility as conflicts over control arise, and perceptions and expectations must be adjusted. Since parents of adolescents must adapt to these changes, rigid or authoritarian patterns of child-rearing, as well as inconsistent care, may exacerbate family conflict. Pelcovitz (1984) categorized adolescent-abusing families into three groups: cases of childhood onset with a history of violence in the family of origin; authoritarian and rigid families with parenting styles characterized by denial of family conflict; and overindulgent families where a pattern of permissive parenting coexists with sporadic violent attempts at control. When abuse occurs during adolescence, it may be more responsive to crisis intervention that focuses on clarifying roles, establishing boundaries, settling conflicts centered around power and control, establishing consistent and flexible styles of parenting, and opening or reestablishing more effective patterns of communication. Abused adolescents who have a history of caring and respectful interactions with their parents will have an easier time becoming motivated in therapy for acute problems.

Long-standing patterns of familial abuse, in which negative and unrewarding family interactions are well established and more resistant to change, are less responsive to crisis intervention and generally require long-term treatment. Probably the greatest difference is the fact that adolescents who have been abused throughout their lives will have many more emotional and behavioral problems, and their parents may be unable or unwilling to make the necessary efforts to effect a positive change. In some cases of long-standing abuse, youngsters may benefit from finally being protected and moved to

a safe and secure environment. (I can't say enough about the negative impact on adolescents of encountering abuse and neglect in out-
of-home care facilities established for their care and protection, and
I encourage clinicians to monitor the quality of care provided to children in institutional settings.) At the same time, unfortunately, youngsters' abilities to trust, feel safe, or be receptive to a new environment
may be greatly endangered. An accurate assessment of whether an
adolescent client is a victim of current or cumulative abuse will allow a clinician to determine relevant therapy goals and formats.

CURRENT (ACUTE) ABUSE

As Chapters One and Two have emphasized, adolescence is a time
of change and transition. Adolescents face the challenges of formulating, defining, or reinforcing values and morals. They are also in the
process of forming their identity and self-concept. They may experiment with a range of behaviors and activities, and may be more
or less vulnerable to peer pressure, parental controls, social demands,
or mass media messages. In particular, adolescents are driven to establish autonomy and personal control, and power struggles with
authority figures (including parents and caretakers) may ensue as they
struggle to make their own decisions, utilize time as they see fit,
or select their own friends and activities.

Coincidentally, parents of adolescents are going through their
own developmental stage. Fisher, Berdie, Cook, and Day (1980)
coined the phrase "middlescence" to describe the stage in which adult
parents of adolescents confront a series of stressful experiences in-
their own lives, including physical changes (e.g., wrinkling, decreased
physical abilities, loss of hair, impaired eyesight); a crises in their
roles as parents, workers, spouses, and/or providers; and new
problems (e.g., role reversal with aging parents or children moving
away from home). Specifically, parents of adolescents may find it
difficult to relinquish their parental roles, because other roles or definitions do not seem achievable. A parent of two teenagers who were
preparing to move away from home stated the problem as follows:

"I honestly don't know what I'm going to do with myself. For 18 years my life has revolved around them, their homework, their after-school activities, their parties and friends. I don't know how I'm going to fill my time when they're not here. It's almost as if I don't know what or who I am except their mother. I don't know how I'm going to let go."

Parents who find the letting-go process difficult may deny impending change. They may continue to expect compliance with their rules, as well as absolute adherence to parental schedules regarding after-school time. If adolescents rebel, which may be appropriate during this developmental stage, parents must learn flexibility and the art of compromise. When parents respond rigidly to their adolescents' fitting objections, power struggles eventuate; if left unresolved, these can escalate into full-blown conflicts. Frustrated or angry parents who feel their control slipping may resort to physical violence.

Jackson W. was an articulate, assertive African-American 16-year-old whom his parents described as "an angel turned warrior" in the last year. A school counselor noted a bruise on the youngster's face and reported the incident to child protective services. After an investigation, the child protective services worker was satisfied that the youngster's injury was an isolated incident, and encouraged the family to receive counseling. Both parents agreed that they had reached their wits' end and sought therapy to get things "back in control." They expressed deep worries about their son's behavior, which they both felt was beyond "normal adolescent troubles." Both parents also compared Jackson to themselves at his age and seemed incredulous about his "rowdy, defiant" behavior.

Mr. W. complained that the school was not backing him up in his attempts to get Jackson's behavior under control. He seemed to have great disdain for the school counselor, who had made the referral to the authorities. "I still don't know how he earns his salary," Mr. W. said about the school counselor. "He doesn't have the slightest idea what we should do. I don't think he has any kids of his own, do you? Because you don't know what it's like unless you've been there."

I empathized with Mr. and Mrs. W., and made some opening remarks about adolescence and how difficult it can be to find the balance between guiding children and letting them find their own way. The following conversation developed:

FATHER: My philosophy is quite simple: As long as he's living in my house, eating my food, and sleeping under my roof, he's got to follow my rules.

THERAPIST: Basically, I agree with you. Jackson is living under your roof and must adhere to your rules.

FATHER: I hear a "but" coming on.

THERAPIST: Well, more like an "and." And, at the same time, I think it's important to give Jackson a chance to make some of his own decisions, so he can start preparing himself for living on his own.

MOTHER: Well, we've still got a little time before that happens.

THERAPIST: Oh? Isn't he a junior now?

MOTHER: Yes, but he hasn't even started talking about what he's gonna do after high school.

FATHER: Well, he has mentioned junior college to me.

MOTHER: I didn't know that.

THERAPIST: What's your reaction?

MOTHER: Well, I guess that's good. Did he say where he was looking?

FATHER: He mentioned Montgomery Junior College.

MOTHER: But that's so far away.

FATHER: Not too bad, a bus ride.

MOTHER: I guess so.

THERAPIST: How do you feel about Jackson talking about moving away?

FATHER: Well, nobody's said anything about moving away. He might stay at home and take the bus to the Montgomery.

THERAPIST: And he might also be planning to move out after senior year.

FATHER: He hasn't mentioned that at all.

THERAPIST: And your reaction?

FATHER: To what? To his not talking to me about that?

THERAPIST: Yes.

FATHER: Well, I don't know. I think it probably means he's not thinking of going anywhere any time soon, although . . .

THERAPIST: Although?

FATHER: Although the way we're getting on right now, I wouldn't blame him if he wanted to leave.

THERAPIST: How come?

FATHER: Well, we just seem to get into it all the time. It's been really difficult lately.

THERAPIST: Give me an example of the kind of things you get into.

FATHER: Tonight's a perfect example, isn't it? (*Looking at Mrs. W.*) He knew we were coming here, he knew when to be home, and he didn't show up on time. We tried calling to find out where he was, what he was doing, but nobody had seen him. Then I wonder, "Where is he? What's he doing?" And I get really hot. When we get home, I'm sure we'll get into a major blowout.

THERAPIST: Describe a major blowout.

FATHER: Loud, lots of obscenities, lots of back and forth . . .

THERAPIST: Do you get anything settled?

FATHER: Hell, no.

THERAPIST: How do you feel about these blowouts?

FATHER: It's not good. It's not good.

THERAPIST: What do you think, Mrs. W.?

MOTHER: I think Dwayne is too hard on Jackson. I think he still wants him to be a little boy who prefers to be with his father no matter what his friends are doing.

FATHER: (*To Mrs. W.*) You know what his friends are doing?

MOTHER: No, I don't. I don't know what they're doing. I know you suspect them of being bad kids, but I don't know if that's so.

FATHER: You know what they look like – street hoods. You know they smoke and drink.

MOTHER: You used to smoke and drink when you were his age.

FATHER: Yeah, but not with a bunch of hoods.

THERAPIST: Let me back up a second, if you don't mind. Your wife says that she thinks you want Jackson to stay a little boy, not grow up, still be your little boy. What do you think about that?

FATHER: Well, somewhat that's true. I miss our fishing trips, and going out for burgers together. I admit that. But I also want him to grow up and be a fine, productive youngster, not get involved in all that self-pitying street behavior – you know, the kids with the chips on their shoulders.

THERAPIST: So you see him in transition now.

FATHER: Yes.

MOTHER: Yes.

THERAPIST: And your job is to guide him through this transition from boy to man.

FATHER: If I don't kill him first. (*Laughter*)

THERAPIST: I know what you mean. Sometimes you get so frustrated and angry you think you might actually obliterate him.

FATHER: Well, I didn't mean that literally. It was just a joke.

THERAPIST: I know, but jokes sometimes carry hidden meaning.

FATHER: Not here.

THERAPIST: The reason I mention that is that I'm wondering if you ever feel that you get out of control with Jackson. You've talked about blowouts, and escalations, and fights. Has it ever gotten physical?

MOTHER: That's what worries me the most – that Jackson will haul off and hit his father back.

THERAPIST: What do you mean, hit him back?

MOTHER: When his dad uses the belt on him, I worry that Jackson is going to fight back one of these days.

THERAPIST: So the fights with Jackson do get physical?

FATHER: On occasion. But it's not like I beat him or anything. Mostly I use the belt to scare him, and I hit a chair or wall to make my point.

THERAPIST: Have you ever hit him hard enough to leave marks on his body?

FATHER: Only one time.

THERAPIST: When was that?

FATHER: About 6 months ago. He turned toward me when I was swinging the belt, and I got him with the buckle on the side of his face.

THERAPIST: So he had a mark on his face?

FATHER: He had swelling and a mark.

THERAPIST: How'd you feel about that?

FATHER: I felt bad about it on the one hand, and on the other, I thought, "Well, maybe now he'll pay attention to what I say."

THERAPIST: Has he?

FATHER: Has he what?

THERAPIST: Has he paid more attention since that time you hit him on the face?

FATHER: No.

THERAPIST: What do you think, Mrs. W.?

MOTHER: I think he's more angry than ever now.

THERAPIST: You mean since Mr. W. hit him on his face with the belt?

MOTHER: Yeah, he talked about his face for weeks.

THERAPIST: Saying what?

MOTHER: How it hurt, how it was swollen, how kids had asked him what happened. Things like that.

THERAPIST: So it probably wasn't effective as a teaching tool.

MOTHER: That's what I think. I think it made things worse.

FATHER: I don't know about that. But yeah, I don't think it helped anything. And . . . never mind.

THERAPIST: You sure?

FATHER: I did feel badly about hurting him.

THERAPIST: Parents often feel remorse when they feel they've hurt their children.

FATHER: He's just so darn frustrating.

THERAPIST: You feel like you don't know what to do next.

FATHER: That's why we're here.

THERAPIST: Well, I have some ideas, which you may or may not be willing to try.

FATHER: We're game if you can tell us what to do.

THERAPIST: My guess is that you need to communicate with each other, listening to each other's different perspectives. When was the last time you really listened to Jackson's perspective on things?

FATHER: I try to listen, but sometimes he's so thick-headed.

THERAPIST: So you try . . . how effective do you feel?

FATHER: Not too much right now.

THERAPIST: How about you, Mrs. W.?

MOTHER: Well, I've always felt pretty good about listening to him, but the problem is that he doesn't seem to be talking to us any more.

THERAPIST: Since when?

MOTHER: Last 2 years or so, there's been a big change.

THERAPIST: That would be right on time. Adolescence is a time when kids really keep things to themselves a lot, or they confide mostly in their friends. Parents often feel clueless, left out.

MOTHER: I miss our talks.

THERAPIST: You miss your talks together, and your husband misses his time alone with his son. Again, this is typical of how parents feel when their kids are going through adolescence. It's funny, people always talk about the kids going through this stage of development, but the truth is that everyone around them goes through it with them. You're all going through adolescence.

FATHER: And this time it's worse than my original time.

THERAPIST: Your adolescence was easy?

FATHER: Relatively speaking. Those were easier times in many ways, not as many temptations, not as much anger and violence in the world.

THERAPIST: And it sounds like you were close to your family, and found it easy to do what they asked.

FATHER: That's really changed in this day and age. We never thought to question our parents or talk back. We respected our parents. That's not how it is any more. Not only Jackson – some of our friends have even worse problems with their kids.

THERAPIST: So you both had an easier time in your adolescence.

MOTHER: Well, not me as much. I loved my parents, still do, but there was never a closeness between us, so I remember being really lonely. I was a lonely, kind of sad young girl. Didn't trust many people.

THERAPIST: Yep. Kids have lots of different experiences, and feeling alone, lonely, or sad is certainly one of the experiences I hear about the most.

FATHER: So, Doctor, what do you suggest we do?

THERAPIST: Well, I'd like to start today with an experiment, a contract, and an invitation.

FATHER: All right.

THERAPIST: The experiment is about today and the fact that he didn't get home in time to come to the appointment with you. What I want you to do is to experiment with a new behavior. Ordinarily, it sounds like you'd go home and "get into it" with him for not being on time, right?

FATHER: Yes. We'd go back and forth about breaking commitments.

THERAPIST: What I'd like you to do today is to go home, and go about your business until Jackson says something to you about being late. When he does, simply tell him that it was too bad he couldn't make it, that you thought it was a good meeting, that you learned a lot about youngsters, and that you are looking forward to the next visit. Then hand him this card, with my phone number and name, and tell him to call me to make an appointment whenever it's convenient to him and doesn't interfere with his busy schedule. If he asks a lot of questions, give brief answers, monosyllabic answers – "Yes," "No," "Okay," – and change the topic of conversation.

FATHER: Well, that's a change of pace. What if he never mentions it?

THERAPIST: Well, wait a while to make sure he has enough time to bring it up himself. If he doesn't, then make a brief statement to him including that you went to the therapy session, you liked it, you learned a lot about youngsters, and you're looking forward to returning. Then hand him my card, and be sure you tell him that I'd like him to call me when it's convenient to him, given his busy schedule. Then we'll see what happens. By the way, don't ask him if he's called, and don't remind him to do so.

FATHER: Okay.

MOTHER: Hm . . . we'll see if we can do this.

THERAPIST: That was the experiment. Now for the contract. I would like us to make a verbal contract that you won't hit Jackson with a belt, your hand, or anything else. I will be teaching you how to diffuse arguments rather than escalate them, and I will be helping the three of you reestablish more positive contact with each other. Sounds like right now, the bulk of your interactions are negative and unrewarding. So you both are missing more rewarding interactions with Jackson. My guess is if you're missing the more positive contact, he is too.

FATHER: Sure, this isn't a real problem with us anyway.

THERAPIST: Good. Then it shouldn't be that hard for you to keep your end of the contract. And lastly, the invitation. I'd like to invite you to make a list of Jackson's positive and negative behaviors – the things you do and don't have trouble with. I'm inviting you to find or rediscover those things about Jackson that you're already satisfied with. At some later point, it will be important for us to meet together and begin to review some of these things.

MOTHER: So you will want to see us together?

THERAPIST: Yes, although now that I've seen you alone and gotten your side of the story, I would like to hear Jackson's side of the story.

FATHER: He'll talk your head off, probably. He can be so charming to outsiders.

MOTHER: (Laughter) He does like to talk. Just not to us.

THERAPIST: And you both seem proud of the fact that he's articulate.

MOTHER: He's like his dad that way.

As the dialogue above makes clear, Mr. and Mrs. W. reported sudden conflicts with their child, which seemed specifically related to the fact that they had difficulty with their son's autonomy. As Jackson chose to spend time away from home, became secretive and uncommunicative, and seemed reluctant to volunteer his current ideas or plans, his parents felt concerned about losing their son. This concern was communicated to Jackson via criticisms and conflicts surrounding his friends, curfews, and academic performance. The more Jackson focused away from his parents, the more his parents sought to control him. My treatment with this family consisted of encouraging the parents to allow Jackson to make more of his own decisions, so he could learn from his mistakes. I facilitated discussion of curfews, so that Jackson could negotiate what he believed to be fair and age-appropriate; I also instructed the parents to share information about themselves, rather than engaging in an interview format, which was quite unsuccessful with Jackson. Because this family had a strong foundation of love, respect, and positive emotional contact in the past, there was a reservoir of positive feelings from which to draw. The family responded well to interventions designed to minimize the negative contacts and maximize the positive, rewarding exchanges that they had previously enjoyed.

In this particular case, Jackson's adolescence and his parents' inability to loosen their control had contributed to unresolvable conflicts, which had escalated to physical violence. The violence, however, had surfaced during recent interactions and did not have a long-standing history. Mr. and Mrs. W. had a background of parental successes, and my job was to help them reclaim the positive interactive patterns they had employed in the past. This was a very different scenario from that encountered with families of adolescents in which the abuse has been chronic.

Whereas the W. family presented in treatment with conflicts that resulted in physical violence, situations of sexual abuse, emotional abuse, or neglect can also arise during a youngster's adolescence, as in the case of Jennifer S. Jennifer, a European-American girl, was sexually approached by her father when she turned 14, and she was sexually abused until she ran away at age 17. She disclosed the sexual abuse at a shelter for runaway youths, and a medical exam revealed two sexually transmitted diseases. The police charged Mr. S. with two counts of sodomy, and he served 6 months in prison and was required to attend therapy.

During the initial assessment, Mr. S. exhibited partial denial: Although he admitted being sexual with Jennifer (fondling her and "letting her" masturbate him), he denied having intercourse with her, and he blamed the sexual abuse on Jennifer. My reconstructed memory of his early statement went something like this:

"This kid is hot to trot; she has been for years. As far back as I can remember, she was a tease. She wore skimpy clothes; she was always jumping on me and wanting to touch me and kiss me. When she was little, I thought she was a pest and she'd get over it, but she never did. As you can see, she's kind of well endowed and has been since she was 12. She asked me to buy her a bra. Her mother was never home and didn't take much of an interest in her. I could see she was looking like a slut, so I took her to buy a bra. I guess this is when I first noticed that she was coming on to me. She wanted me to come in and 'help her' try on her bras. We were in this little tiny room together and there she was, flashing her tits at me and making me touch her. I remember clearly that she bent down and asked me to pull her boobs up, if you know what I mean [he gestured]. I got kind of uncomfortable and left, and she got mad at me and pouted all the way home because I didn't want to stay in the dressing room with her."

Mr. S. denied that there were sexual problems with Jennifer prior to her adolescence, and insisted that what he described as her "womanly desires" wore him down to the point where he was unable to resist. Treatment efforts were marginally successful with Mr. S., who remained convinced that he had fallen prey to a conniving woman-child. He insisted that no one else would ever understand what he had seen and experienced with his daughter, and could not fathom how he was being held accountable for what he believed were his daughter's "sins of the flesh."

As Mr. S.'s statement suggests, he apparently had a history of being troubled by his child's requests for physical affection. When she was little, he saw these requests as a nuisance; however, when the child developed overt signs of womanhood, he projected inappropriate sexual motivation and perceived her to be seductive with him. Instead of setting sexual limits on the youngster (e.g., instructing Jennifer to try on her bra alone or get help from a saleslady, if in fact she had asked him for help in the dressing room), he began to respond to her as if he were being seduced in reality. He perceived her intent as sexual, even though Jennifer would later report to me that she was simply trying to get her dad to notice her and give her positive attention.

Jennifer described a lonely childhood in which her parents were emotionally and physically unavailable to her. "I can't ever remember either Mom or Dad just holding me, or giving me a kiss good night," she lamented. "My mom was just never home, and my dad would watch TV all the time when he was at home. When I was little, I would try to sit on his lap so he would look at me, but he just wouldn't." Jennifer stated that the only times she got attention from her father were when she wore short skirts or see-through blouses. "He bought me the clothes I wore; he picked them all out," Jennifer stated. "Then he would tell me I looked good enough to eat."

Over time, Mr. S. became obsessed with Jennifer's appearance, encouraging her to wear provocative clothing, and asking her to go shopping with him so she could model clothes for him. He proudly described an occasion in which he had been at a department store with Jennifer while she tried on clothes, and some young men gathered around to watch Jennifer model skimpy nightwear, commenting to him how lucky he was to have such a hot girlfriend. Mr. S. was quite taken with the notion that others might think Jennifer was his girlfriend, and encouraged the men to stay and watch how sexy she could really look with the wardrobe he had picked out for her. Jennifer reported that when she complained to her father about the men watching her, he told her to be grateful that men found her attractive at all, since she had "massive thighs."

In this particular case, Mr. S. developed an inappropriate sexual attraction to his daughter, whom he simultaneously praised and criticized. His sexual preoccupation eventually became aggressive behavior, replete with cognitive distortions in which he would hold her accountable for his sexual transgressions. A number of factors contributed to the emergence of sexual abuse in this family, including Jennifer's longing for parental affection, her mother's physical and emotional unavailability, and Mr. S.'s projection of inappropriate sexual intent to his daughter, coupled with his inability to alter his abusive sexual behaviors. It is interesting to note that although this father was emotionally distant from this youngster, the overt signs of her sexuality during adolescence were what precipitated his interest in her.

Sammy F. was a 15-year-old Hispanic boy who appeared depressed and isolated in school. A teacher referred him to therapy when Sammy's macabre drawings caught his attention. When the teacher asked Sammy about his drawings, the themes of death and dying were unsettling: Every picture had someone who was being buried, had body parts sawed off, or was bleeding to death in an alley or back road.

During therapy, Sammy gleefully made picture upon picture of catastrophic situations in which someone's life was compromised. And in every picture the person (almost always a man) whose life was threatened was alone, isolated, and desolate, with no one to care whether he lived or died.

A psychiatric evaluation confirmed Sammy's major depressive episode and suicidality. A social history uncovered that his father had been an alcoholic who fell and hit his head, bleeding to death in an alley on his way home. Sammy was 12 at the time of his father's death, and his brother Billy was 6. The mother apparently viewed Sammy as capable of taking care of himself, and focused her concern and caretaking on her younger son. Sammy was told that he was now the "man of the family," and his mother demanded his participation as a caretaker to Billy and a companion to herself.

The mother plunged into work in order to support herself and her two children. Sammy was often alone taking care of Billy. He learned to put Billy in front of the television and withdrew to go to his own room to draw. When the mother came home she took care of Billy, and sometimes forgot to come into the bedroom to say hello or good night to Sammy. The family organized into a specific constellation of Billy and the mother in a primary relationship, and Sammy as an outsider, who often stayed home alone as his mother and brother went shopping, to the movies, or to the park. It was as if the mother only had energy for her younger child, whom she perceived as still needing her, and could not find room in her heart for Sammy, whom she viewed as distant and independent. Coincidentally, Sammy had been very close to his father; he was named for him and looked very much like him. Strangers would sometimes ask him if he was Samuel F.'s son because the resemblance was so strong. It is possible that the mother withdrew from Sammy because he reminded her so much of her dead husband. Nevertheless, her rationale about why she did not attend to him was clear: "He's a young man now, capable of taking care of himself." His adolescence was perceived as a signal of his independence, regardless of the reality of the situation. In fact, Sammy was a deeply lonely child who missed his father tremendously and had developed an obsession with death. In his drawings, this preoccupation was at the forefront; they indicated a sense of tremendous guilt at not rescuing his father, who had bled to death while Sammy slept comfortably in his bed.

Treatment with this family included helping the mother and both sons to grieve for the father's death. I encouraged the family members to talk together about their memories of the father, and to allow themselves both to express their sad feelings and to comfort each other. The mother was initially resistant to following these directives, finding it painful and disturbing to talk about her dead husband; however, she eventually realized that her sons both harbored feelings of guilt about their father's death, as she did also.

I also facilitated contact between Sammy and his mother, helping her to see Sammy as a lonely and sad child who had lost his father at a very important developmental phase, and needed his mother's attention and caretaking. She slowly began viewing him less as an independent and self-sufficient young man, and more as a tall child who needed comfort and attention from his mother and who benefited from feeling a sense of belonging to his family.

Once the mother and Sammy were able to talk about their guilt for sleeping through Mr. F.'s death, Sammy's preoccupation with death waned. The first drawing he made that did not include a dying person was a picture of himself, his brother, and his mother, cooking a barbecue outdoors.

As all three of these case examples indicate, something about adolescence itself may elicit specific reactions from parents. Parental misperceptions or fears must be acknowledged and addressed, and parental controls must be relinquished when they contribute to conflictual interactions and power struggles that are left negatively unresolved. Premature loosening of control (contact) must also be addressed.

CUMULATIVE (CHRONIC) PATTERNS OF ABUSE

As mentioned previously, my clinical experience has shown me that a long-standing pattern of ongoing, cumulative abuse, in which negative child-rearing patterns persist into adolescence, is more likely to be resistant to clinical intervention. I have found that these patterns of negative child rearing often escalate as youngsters develop coping strategies (or symptoms), such as running away, sexual compulsions, aggressive or violent behavior, substance use, or reliance on defiant or retaliatory behavior. Indeed, M. B. Straus (1994) points out that "delinquency, running away, truancy, drug and alcohol use, schizophrenia, prostitution, teen pregnancy,[1] juvenile homicide, parricide, and suicide have all been associated with abuse of adolescents" (p. 108). As Krystal (1978) has noted, adolescents attempt to fend off the fear of being overwhelmed through symptom formation, which McDougall (1982–1983) describes as the adolescents' attempt to "self-cure" the traumatic state.

Ideally, abusive or neglectful patterns can be identified and stopped early in a child's developmental process. However, if inappropriate or unsafe caretaking behaviors become long-standing patterns of interaction, adolescents are chronically revictimized and suffer from the cumulative impact of continual maltreatment.

In Chapter One, research findings related to the impact of child abuse have been discussed, as have mitigating variables and resiliency. The most important conclusion is that each abused child "ex-

---

[1] A recent study (Boyer, 1995) found that 62% of pregnant adolescents had experienced contact molestation, attempted rape, or rape prior to their first pregnancy. Although no direct causal link is implied, it does appear childhood sexual abuse and sexual exploitation are factors in adolescent high-risk sexual behavior and pregnancy. In addition, although reports of incest pregnancy are mentioned sporadically in the literature, the possibility of such pregnancy exists and should be carefully assessed.

periences disruptions in areas and ways unique to him or her" (McCann et al., 1988, p. 79). Culley and Flanagan (1995) caution against seeing the impact of abuse as static, since "sometimes the meaning of the event is changed to a traumatic one by maturation and development" (p. 19) or by an increased capacity for cognitive reassessment. Kegan (1982) theorizes that children will actively work on their understanding of the victimization.

Perhaps one of the reasons why abuse throughout childhood taxes youngsters' resources is that there is little opportunity for progressive age-appropriate exposure to tolerable amounts of stimulation, which might offer the child an opportunity to build immunity (Edgcumbe & Gavshon, 1985). Given that maltreated children are relentlessly exposed to difficult and painful experiences, their affective regulation is jeopardized, as is their self-regulation of thoughts and behaviors. Clearly, some youngsters who face overwhelming experiences during childhood employ a variety of defenses including denial, dissociation, repression, suppression, and splitting. Depending on the frequency and level of reliance on these defensive strategies, adolescents may be unable or unwilling to integrate their chaotic or painful childhoods, and may instead engage in behavioral reactivity or self-destructive behaviors. These, in turn, may elicit attention from others and precipitate a referral for treatment.

One of the most critical factors in mitigating the impact of abuse is protection. Identification of child abuse often leads to an investigation designed to ascertain whether it is possible for a child to be safe in his or her home environment. When abuse is interrupted by transferring the child to a safe physical environment, or by helping parents or other caretakers design a safe environment, the child may learn that abuse is unacceptable and that he or she is worth protecting.

Unfortunately, children who live in situations of chronic abuse receive neither the protection nor the subsequent sense of worthiness that might help their perception of their fates. If the abuse continues unabated, its lessons are insidious: Children inevitably blame themselves for being abused and hold themselves, rather than their parents or other trusted figures, accountable. Small children in particular are prone to evaluate the situation vis-à-vis their own status, evaluating whether it is the abusers or themselves who are "bad." Understandably, young children protect the figures they idealize, and blame themselves for the abuse they incur at the hands of caretakers. Even when children grow older and may view the situation more realistically, or even shift the blame to the abusers, they may continue to have underlying worries or concerns about whether or not they have attained love. It is this continual struggle to be loved and accepted by abusive figures that becomes a major contributing factor in adolescent development and the completion of the developmental tasks of adolescence. Unfortunately, chronically abused children believe there is something wrong with them, have few expectations of themselves or others, and may sometimes behave in ways that elicit confirmation of their negative self-views. Abused adolescents make the physical transition into adolescence without a smooth parallel emotional transition. As these youngsters concede and acquiesce, negotiating survival skills on a day-to-day basis, the emotional resources allocated for developmental tasks are depleted.

Adolescents with a history of chronic abuse also develop cognitive abilities that allow them to discern and reevaluate their past experiences, and yet these cognitions are influenced by earlier perceptions that may have become belief systems. For example, if a boy of 8 perceives his abuse as stemming from something about him that he views as inherently defective, he may establish a belief system that he "got what he deserved," and may continue to believe that there is something basically wrong with him. Similarly, a girl who is neglected may believe that she is simply not lovable. I've often heard people who were hurt by their parents say, "It wasn't their fault; they did the best they could. I was just no good from the get-go." Sexually abused children may assume responsibility by citing their inability to say "no," their not telling anyone, or their having physical pleasure. They use this evidence to support their belief that something wrong, defective, or inappropriate about them caused their abuse. (See examples in Chapter Five.)

Still other children learn another strong lesson of abuse: No matter what they do or say, they cannot stop the abuse from happening, since they do not have personal power or control. They may there-fore think of themselves as vulnerable and helpless, since they are unable to effect necessary changes. This type of thinking is problemat-ic for adolescents, who evaluate themselves harshly – forgetting that their very dependency on, lack of power over, and love for the abusers all compromise their ability to stop the abuse.

As youngsters mature and develop cognitively, they may recog-nize more options or opportunities. They may also develop addi-tional coping strategies, some healthier than others. Some adolescents who used the defensive strategy of dissociation, which allowed them to make emotional escapes from immediate pain, may now turn to alcohol to effect a similar kind of emotional and physical numb-ness. Adolescents may also turn to others for the affection and at-tention they lack at home; unfortunately, these youngsters may not be well versed in self-protection and may put themselves in harm's way. Their judgment may also be impaired by emotional problems regarding their self-esteem and self-worth. Youngsters who believe that they do not deserve positive attention may bargain for nega-tive attention instead, by being provocative or uncooperative. Young-sters who feel unsafe may gravitate toward unsafe situations, perhaps wanting to test their own sense of mastery and control. Individuals abused early in life are often revictimized later. This correlation may exist as a result of low self-esteem, cognitive distortions about them-selves and their futures, and aborted attempts to achieve a sense of control and mastery. In addition, some children cannot protect them-selves because they suffer from learned helplessness, which affects their abilities to say "no" or take action on their own behalf.

Yet another important lesson of familial child abuse stems from the fact that the violence, inattention, or sexual exploitation occurs in the context of an intimate, theoretically loving relationship. A child who is hurt by someone outside the family can return to a safe and appropriate environment where he or she is believed, com-forted, and taken for appropriate medical or psychological attention if needed. A child who is hurt by a family member views the fami-ly environment as potentially dangerous, with varying degrees of secrecy, loyalty conflicts, and confusion. It is particularly difficult for abused children to perceive or understand their abuse when it comes from a trusted and loved person, in whom there is a personal investment, including (but not limited to) personal survival. The child's dependency on familial relationships for love, acceptance, guidance, and maintenance of physical needs jeopardizes the child's ability to view the situation realistically and hold the abuser accountable.

Adolescents with chronic abuse are likely to be most susceptible to negative consequences of abuse if they have been unable to complete developmental tasks, and if they hold themselves culpable in their victimization. Their inability to protect themselves as young children leaves them feeling vulnerable, helpless, and rageful as they mature; eventually, they may strive to discard their sense of helplessness in favor of an aggressive and controlling stance toward others.

Jason L. was a 16-year-old Native American youth referred to group treatment for sexually molesting an 8-year-old girl. His primary therapist shared his cultural heritage and addressed his feelings of isolation from the Native tribal life he had discarded when he ran away from the reservation after years of physical abuse.

Jason was a quiet, compliant youngster whose temper flared up when he was confronted with adversity, particularly by same-sex peers. The group experience provided him with stimuli that provoked his wrath on a weekly basis. Although he protested loudly to his own therapist, Jason was attentive and cooperative in group sessions unless someone teased him or challenged him directly.

Jason's mother had died at his birth, and his father had been bitter toward Jason thereafter, allowing the maternal grandmother to assume primary caretaking responsibility. Jason's father gradually developed a serious alcohol problem and would leave the reservation for longer and longer periods of time, often being picked up on street corners and taken to jail for vagrancy. Jason's grandmother provided stability until Jason was 4 years of age. However, after she died there was sporadic care from the extended family, and Jason's father belittled the child for his inability to take care of himself and act like a man. Jason described his childhood as lonely; he spent most of his time by himself, either in his own home or outdoors. Other children teased him because he did not engage in peer activities, and since he spent most of his time alone, others did not have the opportunity to get to know him. Jason's father held him responsible for his wife's death and seemed to resent Jason's very existence. Jason reported "trying hard" to please his father, although his father never once seemed grateful or happy. Verbal abuse turned to severe physical abuse when Jason was approximately 6 years of age. Jason then avoided peer activities because he was ashamed that his many bruises would show and become a source of ridicule from others.

Jason remembered a Native American social worker visiting the home and talking with Jason's father. Jason's father confided to her that it had been devastating for him to lose his wife, and that he had lost direction after her death. The social worker spent hours talking with him, and after she left Jason's aunt seemed to come by more frequently, although eventually Jason's father did not welcome her visits. By the time he was 13, Jason was extremely bitter, lonely, and angry; he was undersocialized and had not participated in family or community life in spite of others' attempts to elicit his involvement. This child who had "fallen through the cracks" then broke away from traditional life, vowing never to return. He found his way to Los Angeles, where he lived on the streets. At 15 he was placed in a Native American foster home, after being returned to his reservation three times and running away each time, refusing to live with his "drunk father."

Jason had numerous learning and developmental delays, including speech delays and learning difficulties – understandably so, since he had spent most of his childhood without proper attention or stimulation. Although he had attended school, his quiet demeanor caused his teachers to view him as problem-free. It was only when he became aggressive with his peers and ran away that teachers concerned themselves with him, speculating that it must have been difficult for him to have lost his mother and grandmother. Jason was also very immature, preferring the company of much younger children to that of peers. Given his choice, he would spend his time with children half his age; this may have reflected the developmental stage at which he was most affected by the emotional unavailability of his father, guilt over his mother's death, and the physical beatings, which on some level he believed he deserved for causing his mother's death.

In his foster care placement, he stayed to himself. In spite of efforts to integrate him into the family, Jason assumed his usual position of outsider and loner, with the exception of his interest in the 8-year-old biological daughter of his foster parents. The parents happily observed Jason's interest in the girl, and grew accustomed to his combing her hair for long periods of time and sitting with her while she watched television. They thought he was finally learning to interact with another human being, and felt encouraged to see the two youngsters playing; they were oblivious to the age difference and to Jason's preoccupation with her physical appearance.

However, the little girl, Rosa, eventually told her mother that Jason was tickling her under her dress, and that he had recently taken down her pants to look at her privates. When the mother asked Rosa a few more questions, she discovered that Jason had been showing Rosa his genitals, asking her to touch the soft skin of the penis, and combing her hair while his penis grew erect. Jason was transferred to another foster home as a result of Rosa's disclosure, and his referral to treatment was mandated by the courts, in which he was adjudicated as a sex offender.

Jason showed classic signs of abuse and neglect: pseudomaturity and superficial autonomy; a markedly ill-defined sense of identity; lack of direction (having had woeful lack of guidance); and poor self-esteem, stemming from a view of himself as unworthy of positive attention. When group members or leaders asked him to talk about himself, he was suspicious and reluctant to self-disclose. He was very uncomfortable with attention, especially positive attention; this made it difficult for him to tolerate some of the potentially beneficial aspects of group therapy.

Jason's history had contributed in great part to his sexual acting out. Without appropriate role models or guidance, his sexual development had left him confused and frustrated. His father had beaten him for masturbating when he was young and put his hands in a fire to teach him not to "waste his seed." Because of his social isolation, Jason never developed appropriate interactions with peers of either gender. His feelings of inadequacy and of guilt for causing his mother's death contributed further to his sexual confusion.

His father's physical beatings had also created a sense of helplessness in Jason, with concomitant feelings of rage that were often left unexpressed. His primary defense was to flee uncomfortable or painful situations, and he had never experienced a satisfactory interpersonal relationship. He described feeling closest to his grandmother, but resented the fact that she did not stop the beatings, choosing instead to act as though they never occurred.

Because Jason was so immature and needy, he had found comfort in the nonthreatening relationship offered by Rosa, who accepted him for who he was, looked up to him, and asked him for nothing. He had enjoyed the sensation of combing her hair and dressing her in different clothes, but felt defensive about the sexual arousal he felt toward her.

During one of the group sessions Jason remembered that he had been told his mother had long, smooth hair like Rosa's, and that he sometimes wondered what it would have been like to comb his mother's hair.

SUMMARY AND CONCLUSIONS

As we have seen, adolescents can be abused throughout their childhood and adolescence in either continuous or sporadic fashion. Some abused adolescents have the cumulative impact of chronic histories of abuse, whereas in other cases adolescents are abused primarily because of the developmental stage they are in, or because of rigid or permissive patterns of child rearing.

Adolescence may precipitate anxiety and confusion in adults who are reaching their own midlife stage when their youngsters approach adolescence. The issues of adolescence and those of "middlescence" are parallel: identity, career choices, pressure to form and maintain long-term intimate relationships, autonomy, and choices regarding the future. Some parents may be unable to let go of control issues to accommodate their adolescents' newfound autonomy; power struggles may ensue as parents try their best to impose their influence over youngsters' life decisions, and these struggles may become physical. Other parents are reminded of their own adolescence as they interact with their youngsters, and perhaps become more vigilant as a result of remembering how they were at this age. If parents were unhappy, unpopular, or left with unfulfilled dreams and ambitions, they may consciously or unconsciously push their children in specific directions to gain vicarious pleasure through their accomplishments.

The cognitive, physical, personality, sexual, and moral developmental tasks of childhood and adolescence are monumental at best. Youngsters need support, guidance, encouragement, and safety in order to make a successful transition to maturity. Without safety, consistency, fulfillment of dependency needs, and attainment of love and a sense of belonging, they will struggle to develop a positive sense of identity, attachment, and ego strength. Child abuse greatly hinders the developmental process, and chronic child abuse causes serious concerns for adolescents.

Adolescents who have received appropriate care throughout their childhoods, only to face abuse that emerges during adolescence, also suffer. However, the fact that sufficient attention has been given to critical developmental tasks gives adolescents without previous abuse a more optimistic prognosis, particularly if the crisis brought on by familial adolescent abuse can be successfully resolved within the family system.

Children who have been abused all their lives have not had similar opportunities to achieve physical, emotional, personality, or cognitive development. Chronic abuse may have left them debilitated or impaired. As adolescents, they will have numerous issues to resolve: developmental delays; impaired identities; feelings of insecurity; inability to trust; internalized or externalized anger; and varying degrees of impairment in their abilities to form positive attachments, friendships, or rewarding intimate relationships. At the same time, many of the qualities that clinicians describe as difficult—resistance, oppositionality, manipulation, anger, negative attention-seeking – may be these youngsters' way to assert boundaries, get their needs met, and exert control in ways denied to them previously.

Adolescents have the disadvantage of coming in bigger packages than younger children, and therefore running the risk of being seen as off-putting, threatening, oppositional, or opinionated, rather than assertive and autonomous. Clinicians must constantly address their countertransference responses to avoid engaging with adolescents in interactional modes reminiscent of their dysfunctional parents. Clinicians must also monitor adolescents' transferential responses and behaviors designed to elicit negative, hostile, or sexualized responses.

CHAPTER FOUR

Assessment and Treatment

ASSESSMENT CONSIDERATIONS

Most adolescents are referred for treatment because their behavior is worrisome or problematic to someone. Although on occasion I have worked with youngsters who seek therapy themselves, this appears to be the exception rather than the rule. Most of the adolescents referred to me have had presenting problems such as sadness or moodiness, self-injury or self-destructive behaviors, substance abuse, suicidal ideation, difficulty making and keeping friends, aggressive behaviors, and/or sexual acting out (including indiscriminate sexual activity or committing sexual offenses). Discussing the emotional and behavioral effects of adolescent physical abuse specifically, Farber and Joseph (1985) found six patterns of reactions: acting out, depression, generalized anxiety, extreme adolescent adjustment problems, emotional–thought disturbance, and helpless dependency. Each reaction led to specific symptomatology. For example, generalized anxiety could result in lack of trust, rationalizing and manipulating, poor concentration, impaired identity development, and academic failure. Many acting-out behaviors may be or have the potential to become life-threatening, such as practicing unsafe sex, becoming substance-dependent, and taking physical risks (e.g., driving under the influence, jumping off bridges, or walking toward traffic on the freeway). Some adolescents become severely depressed and suicidal (internalizing their distress), whereas others become hostile or violent toward others (externalizing it). Finally, parents may bring their youngsters to treatment for a range of problem behaviors that could best be summed up as defiance, oppositionality, isolation, lack of interest in other family members, and negativity. In short, adolescents' symptomatic behaviors can be multiple, varied, and often frightening, and some clinicians stay away from the implied responsibility of trying to help youths who appear so disturbed. Although my clinical experience has been providing outpatient therapy, I often refer youth for psychiatric evaluations to determine suicide or homicide risk, the need for psychopharmacological treatment, as well as situations that require hospitalization. Abused adolescents may benefit from specialized hospital units providing structured inpatient care on issues of prior or current abuse (Cantor, 1995). In addition, referring for psychiatric consultation ensures a team approach, often helpful or necessary in the treatment of abused adolescents.

Children and adolescents are often brought to treatment by parents or caretakers who have abused or neglected them, although these adults rarely announce this at the outset. Every now and then I have been impressed with a parent's ability to engage in self-evaluation, recognize the potential impact of his or her behavior, and show interest in seeking help, no matter what personal cost of embarrassment or shame may ensue. Conversely, I have worked with parents who describe a litany of behaviors that I consider abusive, but that they have normalized as suitable caretaking behaviors.

Many of the symptoms I have listed above occur for reasons other than abuse or neglect, and it is important to approach each case with an open mind about an array of possible contributors. Although this book concerns itself with documented or verified cases of maltreatment by parents or other trusted figures, it is important to note that some adolescents do lie, exaggerate, or fabricate stories about childhood abuse for secondary gains. However, studies addressing the issue of "fictitious allegations of child abuse" indicate that few stories of abuse are fabricated, that these cases occur relatively infrequently, and that when they do occur they are likely to originate in parental coaching, adolescents' attempts to manipulate their circumstances, or children and adolescents suffering from PTSD (Jones & McGraw, 1987). In my experience, when adolescents are lying about childhood abuse, their facts become confused and inconsis-

the possibilities for partnership between treatment and research," (p. 1421), Finkelhor and Berliner (1995) suggest that generic and abuse-specific measures be used together when assessing abused children and adolescents.

Abused adolescents are often perceived as more difficult clients than younger children. When I have asked colleagues to identify the origins of this difficulty, they suggest several factors: Adolescents are resistant; they don't cooperate or comply with treatment; they can be verbally abusive; their range of problem behaviors can appear more pathological than that of younger children; and they are often impulsive. Some colleagues have also confided that adolescents "push their buttons," bringing out a controlling, punitive side of themselves that they don't like. The end result is that those who have difficulty working with adolescents seem to feel frustrated, defeated, and useless – feelings that increase their sense of incompetence in working with this age group. Of course, no one likes feeling incompetent, and some professionals simply work harder to compensate for their feelings of failure; this, in turn, can result in battle fatigue and a lack of enthusiasm about their work.

Many adolescents exhibit a range of problems in miscellaneous settings, including their own homes, foster and group homes, residential treatment centers, schools, and institutional correctional facilities. These youngsters will signal their distress until they are able to relieve some of their pain, confusion, or isolation, and release some of their pent-up affect. It appears that among the most common sources of despair and unhappiness for adolescents are family conflict, neglect, and physical or sexual abuse.

Because most adolescents continue to be in the legal (if not physical) care of their parents, and because their emotional and physical safety is paramount, a comprehensive assessment must include interviews with the entire family. In particular, if the adolescent has been a victim in the past, or has been a victim of out-of-home abuse, the family's ability and willingness to offer support, guidance, and nurturing must be evaluated. The "Guide to Family Observation and Assessment" (Singer et al., 1993) is a very useful conceptual framework for assessing families in a systematic way. Clinicians using this guide will observe and inquire about a number of variables including family "nationalism" (p. 18); involvement; respect; appreciation of developmental needs, abilities, and positive behaviors; parental perceptions of children as a subgroup; generational distinctions; adult/spousal alliance; family communication; family problem-solving and communication skills; family rituals; use of humor and play; domestic violence and substance abuse; sources of family stress; and family involvement with the community. There are other assessment instruments specifically designed for evaluating parent–child interactions and family functioning that might also be helpful in conducting adequate family assessments such as the Parent–Child Relationship Inventory (Gerard, 1994); Parenting Stress Index (Abidin, 1990); and the Family Environment Scale (Moos, 1979).

MY PERSONAL APPROACH TO TREATMENT

My professional persona has been shaped by a great many influences, including things I have read, courses I have attended, teachers, fellow students, and colleagues who have influenced my general approach to treatment through modeling ethical and compassionate clinical work, and my own clinical experience for the past two decades. My clinical experience has been, originally by accident and later by design, skewed: Almost all my clients seek therapy, ordered to do so by the courts, social services or probation departments, as a result of child abuse and neglect. I therefore acknowledge that I am less familiar with problems that do not have their roots in childhood abuse, and this makes me more inclined to find early abuse experiences of great significance in the treatment process.

On the other hand, I have had friends and colleagues (as well as some clients) who seem marginally affected by their abuse experiences, and at times even seem fortified by their early difficulties. The old adage "What doesn't kill you makes you stronger" may be true for some individuals, who manage somehow to balance their abuse experiences by finding ways of overcoming—and, in fact, utilizing—experiences that have been painful, exacting, or temporarily debilitating.

Lastly, it is abundantly clear to me that some people survive by denying the facts or the impact of early childhood abuse. They simply deny these early events, will not discuss them, and make conscious efforts to "forget" that which is unpleasant and no longer in their control. In addition to these individuals who consciously suppress their painful histories, others may instead unconsciously repress information, casting it likewise out of conscious awareness. Probably a clearer way of describing repression is to think of it as dissociated memory that remains fragmented and unassimilated.

Providing treatment to individuals with histories of childhood abuse is therefore complex and challenging, and must be tailored to each individual on a case-by-case basis. Techniques that work with one client may be abysmally ineffective or counterindicated with others. As a clinician, I must remain flexible and open to developing treatment interventions with my clients; interventions must be based on what they report and the insights they achieve in treatment, as well as what I observe and share with them. Therapy is never a rigid plan imposed *on* my clients, but rather consists of an exchange of ideas and suggestions, mutually generated and tested. Its success in each case is evaluated through a client's decrease in symptoms and improved general functioning.

AN INTEGRATED THEORETICAL FOUNDATION

Because abuse and neglect have the potential to harm growing children and adolescents in the numerous ways and dimensions described in this book, a number of theoretical frameworks will provide useful guidance and assistance in formulating treatment plans.

One of the most concise statements I have ever read about the therapeutic role is that offered by Elsa Jones (1991). Jones has captured many of the elements that constitute my therapeutic stance:

> As a therapist, I assume that when someone approaches me for help with the difficulties they [sic] are experiencing these may be linked to factors both in their past and in their present, and may have individual and "internal" components as well as interactional and contextual ones. I assume that there is a looping relation-

ship between action and meaning, so that a change in behavior may well lead to the attribution of different meaning, just as a shift in the assumed meaning of events may lead to changes in behavior. I assume that each individual has resources and strengths, no matter how despairing they may be feeling at the moment of coming to therapy, and that it is my job to help them find access to these, without minimizing the seriousness of the troubles by which they may have been overwhelmed. I also assume that people themselves have a better idea of their own history, values, creative resources, and what solutions are likely to fit for them, than any outsider can ever have, so that the therapist's task is, as it were, to help clients roll obstacles out of their path, but not to point out the route they should be following. At the same time I am aware, on the basis of theory as well as observations in therapy and in my own life, that it is difficult to attain an overview or meta-perspective on one's own situation, so that sitting down to talk with someone else, whether a professional therapist or not, may be necessary in order to begin to look at events, connections, and previously obscured aspects of the patterns of action and relationship that accumulate around "the problem." I therefore assume that I am unlikely to know the answer to the client's dilemmas, but that my systemic curiosity, my technical skills (e.g., in asking circular or hypothetical questions), my respectful search for their own skills and resources, my widening of the area of inquiry to include wider contexts that may previously have been left out of account, my challenge to set ways of thinking, and my attempt to create a safe and containing space in which the unthinkable and unsayable can be expressed, will have the effect of freeing up the client's own ability to explore, to grow, and to resolve dilemmas. . . . In summary, I might say, then, that the therapist's major task is to introduce "news of difference" (Bateson, 1980)—that is, flexibility, complexity, options, different perspectives—into the therapeutic conversation with the client, so that the experience of being stuck and having no choice can change into one feeling freed up to create one's own preferred new ways of relating to self and others. (pp. 7–8)

I find a number of Jones's beliefs and opinions invaluable: her view that current difficulties may be linked to factors in the past and present; her respect for individual, interactional, and contextual contributors; her stress on the relationship between action and meaning; her belief in the individual's creative resources, strengths, and history; the notion that many individuals have the ability to find their own solutions; and her emphasis on the client's ability to grow, explore, and resolve dilemmas. I also value her definition of the therapeutic "job," including the clinician's attempts to help individuals find their own resources and solutions; the efforts to roll obstacles out of clients' path without pointing to specific routes to follow; and the application of therapeutic curiosity and broadening of options so that individuals can empower themselves.

Straus (1988) champions an ecological perspective in the treatment of adolescent abuse. She reminds us practitioners "must have available an array of approaches from which to select the most suitable" (p. 110), and she suggests an understanding of the background characteristics of abusive parents (ontogenic development); the interaction among family members (microsystem); the family's relationship to community and helping agencies (exosystem); and the larger cultural fabric of the individual, family, and community (macrosystem).

With this broader context in mind, I draw from other theoretical frameworks to guide my treatment approach. In particular, I am convinced that child abuse and neglect inherently cause disruptions in attachment, and that these disruptions therefore contribute to relational difficulties. The notion of secure and insecure attachment is aptly described by Bowlby (1969, 1973). Attaining secure attachment is one of the first developmental tasks of childhood, and when this task is not successfully completed, it can cause ongoing difficulties in establishing necessary intimate relationships. In particular, a child who is abused early in life may need to resolve attachment-related issues of trust and dependency; until these are addressed in some fashion, other developmental tasks may remain partially or fully unresolved.

When a clinician is considering an individual's context, various other developmental theories can also provide a deeper understanding of the issues that may need attention and resolution. For example, Erikson's (1963) theory of personality development dovetails nicely with Kegan's (1982) focus on identity and self-formation, and together they provide the theoretical impetus for a focus on the individual's evolving sense of self and identity. Kegan (1982) and Coopersmith (1967) note together that the following elements are critical to the formation of positive identity and self-esteem: feelings of significance and belonging; feelings of virtue; attainment of love; and feelings of personal power, mastery, and control. Unfortunately, all of these are compromised by child abuse and neglect.

Since abused children are by definition victimized, the dominant story they form of their lives is often a "problem-saturated" description that has been reinforced in many ways, "leaving no space for them to perform another story" (Kamsler, 1990, p. 21). Narrative therapy has greatly influenced my thinking in this area, partly because it is so nonpathologizing, but also because it urges specific clinical interventions that provide "news of difference," so that clients can see possibilities for new solutions and new self-narratives. Thus, they can balance or rescript a fuller sense of identity—one that is not "abuse dominated," but rather competency-based.

Trauma theory, particularly as defined by van der Kolk (1987), advances the idea that unresolved trauma can cause behavioral reenactments, compulsive behaviors, PTSD symptoms, and physiological responses that can debilitate individuals or cause global impairment. Terr (1994) defines two types of trauma (Type I and Type II), which require different interventions. Herman (1992) suggests that generic PTSD does not fully coincide with what she terms "complex PTSD," which is experienced by survivors of chronic, repetitive, and severe abuse. Herman contends that many survivors of such prolonged trauma experience polarized sensations of numbing and hyperarousal, and that problem behaviors accompany both types of responses (e.g., internalized behaviors such as depression, and externalized behaviors that may put an individual in harm's way). There is a consensus among clinicians who work with trauma that the traumatic experiences must be brought into conscious awareness and processed, with a goal of integrating the material in a less fragmented manner (Herman, 1992). As Cuffe and Frick-Helms (1995) state, "the trauma-specific phase of treatment should focus on the traumatic aspects of the abuse, allowing expression of affects and working through of traumatic memories" (p. 235). However, trauma-specific treatment must be undertaken with great caution and in a structured, purposeful fashion; it should also not begin until individuals have adequate ego strength and an expanded repertoire of coping strategies.

Because the issue of child abuse or neglect almost invariably emerges within the context of family interactions, it is valuable to use a systemic approach (through one individual client, or with several or all family members present), particularly since each family member is affected by parental maltreatment. Abused children often learn to behave in ways that are designed to make them feel safer (e.g., hitting or threatening people), but that instead elicit more negative responses, which then reinforce their already developed feelings of being unworthy or unacceptable. In addition, it is ineffectual and limited to work with abused children and adolescents without making active efforts to protect young clients when they need protection; to educate abusive families by providing them with alternatives to abuse, neglect, or inappropriate and dangerous sexual violations; to set necessary limits; and to utilize a broader system of community accountability (Gil, 1995).

Because abused adolescents present with such a variety of problem behaviors, cognitive-behavioral strategies are almost always needed to help them correct thinking errors and affective dysregulation which contribute to the emergence and maintenance of problematic behaviors. The major objective of cognitive-behavioral therapy is to help clients gain new perspectives on their problems, correct faulty cognitions, and increase behavioral competencies (Zarb, 1992).

Finally, I find it impossible to deal with the issues presented by abused adolescents without viewing them from feminist, sociological, and multicultural perspectives. The reality from a feminist point of view is that women and children have long-standing histories of being disempowered, and that efforts to afford them with protection when needed have been half-hearted at best. I do fully acknowledge the fact that boys and men are also victimized in Western culture; however, they are not now, nor have they been, victimized or devalued in the proportions that women and children have been exploited throughout history. A sociological perspective acknowledges social norms that allow or condone child abuse and neglect (notably, hundreds of homeless families have existed in the United States for the last 15 years, while we cry out against "street children" in countries such as Thailand or Brazil). And a multicultural perspective means that we must treat abused adolescents within the context of their own culture, and recognize that formal therapy as we know it in the mainstream United States is a foreign concept to many people whose culture does not embrace the mental health care system as a useful resource. We must remain open to strategies that respect differences as well as commonalities among cultures, recognize differing levels of acculturation, and draw upon other cultures' healing practices. We need to embrace what may be built into a specific culture as helpful, rather than imposing strategies that may feel awkward and have limited applicability.

In my own work, I make use of the various theoretical frameworks described above to develop a strong therapeutic relationship that over time can provide a safe, rewarding, corrective, and reparative experience to abused adolescents. I also construct therapeutic tasks designed to help these adolescents obtain more and better feedback from the environment, and I ensure that their sense of self is in the forefront as they learn to self-monitor, self-regulate, and develop behaviors that elicit more positive responses. When it seems appropriate and necessary to do so, I address a clients' trauma-related material in a structured and in-depth way, which is fully described in Chapter Five. Finally, I keep in mind that I may need to become a vocal advocate for my adolescent clients as well as other abused adolescents; I recognize that protection may be necessary, and that a broadened view of community accountability (including legal interventions) may also be necessary.

TREATMENT GOALS

The overriding goal of working with adolescent survivors of childhood abuse is to remove obstacles to their growth and development.

This is accomplished by using a competency-based model (Durrant & Kowalski, 1990) that includes the following specific treatment goals:

1. To address each symptomatic behavior, evaluating its potential usefulness, honoring necessary defenses, and providing alternative responses and symptom substitution.
2. To assess and address problems in developmental transitions, attempting to remove obstacles to growth.
3. To assist youngsters in the process of defining self and identity by providing them with new information, asserting their strengths and resources, and helping them identify and express their thoughts and emotions.
4. To give adolescents ample opportunity to develop a sense of competence and mastery.
5. To allow adolescents to explore the idiosyncratic meaning of past abuse, make cognitive reassessments, and detach themselves from feelings of powerlessness and lack of control.
6. When it is necessary and appropriate to do so, to help youngsters with unresolved trauma process the difficult material, in order to move toward integration and empowerment.
7. To help adolescents make decisions and learn to distinguish between those things they can and cannot control.
8. To provide a corrective and reparative experience by being trustworthy, dependable, and consistent, and providing continuity of care.
9. To advocate for change in the family context, and seek and access resources for emotional and physical protection for young clients when necessary.

These treatment goals may be met in numerous ways and by using various creative strategies. The next section presents a number of strategies and techniques that I have found useful in the process of working with adolescent survivors of childhood abuse.

SPECIFIC TREATMENT
STRATEGIES AND TECHNIQUES

Decoding a Symptom and Understanding Its Value/Helpfulness

I have always found it useful to decode symptoms – that is, to attempt to find the creativity and resourcefulness conveyed through a young client's behavior. Even a particularly distressing behavior, such as an adolescent's setting a fire in his or her bedroom, may be viewed as a cry for help. The metaphor of a fire, with the potential to burn out of control or destroy the environment, may be viewed as the youngster's plea for limits and safety. The response must include both the setting of limits ("It is not acceptable for you to do this – we will check your room and clothes for matches every day, you will be grounded for a week, and you will research and write a paper on the danger of fires") and the provision of additional safety and attention ("We need to talk about how to be more helpful to you with your concerns and worries about yourself – we will be spending more time with you, helping you with your homework, or just talking together before you go to sleep").

Some inquiry must be directed at the potential benefits or advantages gained through the symptomatic behavior. For example, Marcia was a 14-year-old referred for self-injury. When I asked her what happened before, during, and after the cutting, she described feeling relieved and safe after she cut her arms. When I asked Marcia to say more about her relief, she stated, "Well, like, finally I just had to feel the pain on my arms, and when I felt that, I didn't feel sad any more." I pointed out to her that it sounded as if it was easier for her to feel physical pain rather than emotional pain. She responded, "Oh, yeah. I get really scared when I'm sad that I might try to kill myself." Her cutting behavior, in paradoxical form, kept her safe from hurting herself. Once we were able to identify the usefulness of the symptom, it was easier to devise a plan (1) to provide an alternative behavior for avoiding painful or scary feelings; and (2) to begin to deal with the sadness in a way that didn't overwhelm her, by having her engage in incremental exposure that would allow her to build tolerance.

Connecting the Dots: Looking at How Past Lessons Influence Current Problems

How do past experiences influence or shape current functioning? In part, it has to do with how children learn through observing or participating in life situations and interactions with significant primary caretakers. If a child grows up in a family in which violence is the status quo, the child is learning not only about how people interact with each other, but also about family and gender roles, conflict resolution, love and affection, and power differentials. The child is also developing expectations about the future, as well as belief systems about reality. For example, a child who knows that violence is an organizing principle within intimate relationships may expect violence to be intertwined with his or her relationships. One abused child confided, "People who love you hurt you," and in that brief sentence summed up his life experience and his expectations about change. He was a child who acted out in school, eliciting negative behaviors from teachers and caretakers. Because he believed that he would be hurt by those who cared, he provoked his caretakers until they acted in familiar ways that reaffirmed and solidified his belief system. Unable to trust, he anxiously awaited or negotiated the next assault – not because he wanted or enjoyed physical pain, or wanted to feel vulnerable, but because he genuinely believed that his fate was predetermined. For him to alter this firm belief system, he had to have a corrective experience: Someone who cared for him would not injure him, even when relentlessly provoked.

"Connecting the dots" is a familiar activity to most children. It consists of drawing lines from one dot to another on a piece of paper until a clearly identified picture seems miraculously to appear. I often offer this metaphor to adolescents who are trying to clarify their feelings and thoughts about their backgrounds. Facts become dots. Reviewing the significant facts of their life and making associations between past and present events (i.e., the lessons learned and carried forward) can provide them with new understanding and increased insight. Here's an example of this process with a youngster who was left to fend for himself starting at age 7:

ADOLESCENT: You don't understand. They bug me all the time. They treat me like I was a kid. I don't need that. I've been taking care of myself forever. They're a day late and a dollar short.

THERAPIST: You remember that time we talked about connecting the dots?

ADOLESCENT: Yeah, vaguely.

THERAPIST: Okay, I'm sure as I tell you about it a little more now, your memory will become more clear. Remember that I said that sometimes there are connections between past and present?

ADOLESCENT: Yeah.

THERAPIST: And that we might not be able to see those right away?

ADOLESCENT: Yeah.

THERAPIST: Okay. Now I'd like you to see what you think is the connection between the trouble you're having with your foster parents right now, and what happened when you were a child.

ADOLESCENT: Nobody was around when I was growing up.

THERAPIST: Your mom kind of left you on your own a lot.

ADOLESCENT: When I was about 7, she was never home. She slept away from the house a lot, and she thought that I was smart enough and brave enough to stay home alone.

THERAPIST: And were you?

ADOLESCENT: Damn straight I was.

THERAPIST: And what else were you?

ADOLESCENT: What do you mean?

THERAPIST: Well, you were brave and smart, and what else?

ADOLESCENT: Nothing else . . .

THERAPIST: Do you remember what you looked like at that age?

ADOLESCENT: I was little. I remember that, because kids used to make fun of me.

THERAPIST: And how did you feel about that?

ADOLESCENT: It made me mad.

THERAPIST: And what else?

ADOLESCENT: I don't know . . . made me feel like there was something wrong with me.

THERAPIST: Okay, so in addition to being smart and brave, you were also a small kid, who sometimes got angry when kids made fun of his size and at other times felt like there was something wrong with him.

ADOLESCENT: Yeah.

THERAPIST: And what else?

ADOLESCENT: Well, I just remember feeling alone, lonely maybe. I looked out the window and everybody else was doing something with somebody, but I was locked in all by myself.

THERAPIST: So when you were a kid you were smart, brave, and angry. You felt different sometimes, and felt lonely too.

ADOLESCENT: Yeah, I guess so.

THERAPIST: Well, that's what you've told me so far.

ADOLESCENT: Yeah.

THERAPIST: And how did you feel about your mom being gone?

ADOLESCENT: I didn't care.

THERAPIST: So sometimes you didn't care. How did you feel the rest of the time?

ADOLESCENT: I don't know. I was mad, I guess – mad that I didn't get to do anything and I had to be locked up all the time.

THERAPIST: And what was your mom doing?

ADOLESCENT: Hah. Who knows? She never clued me in.

THERAPIST: So you didn't know why she was away so much.

ADOLESCENT: She had boyfriends, I know that.

THERAPIST: And she preferred to be with them?

ADOLESCENT: Who cares? I could take care of myself just fine. I didn't need her.

THERAPIST: And you haven't needed anybody since, have you?

ADOLESCENT: No. I don't even know why I just can't be on my own.

THERAPIST: Remember the last time you ran away, where you ended up?

ADOLESCENT: Yeah, but that was just a fluke. It won't happen again.

THERAPIST: Well, I hope not, but one of the reasons you live with adults is so they can watch out for you. It's not always safe on the street, as you found out.

ADOLESCENT: I know, I know.

THERAPIST: So do you remember how you felt before you started feeling like you didn't care about your mom?

ADOLESCENT: Not much.

THERAPIST: Because I imagine that a 3-year-old or 4-year-old would find it hard not to have his mom around?

ADOLESCENT: I don't remember much about that.

THERAPIST: Any memories about you and your mom early on?

ADOLESCENT: The only thing I remember is that once she took me to a merry-go-round and it was just her and I, and she bought me cotton candy, and I sat next to her on a big horse and she held my hand even when the horses went up and down.

THERAPIST: And she never let go?

ADOLESCENT: Well, when it was over.

THERAPIST: But I mean while you were on the merry-go-round?

ADOLESCENT: Right.

THERAPIST: And how did that feel?

ADOLESCENT: Good (*mumbling*).

THERAPIST: I'm sorry, I didn't hear.

ADOLESCENT: It felt good.

THERAPIST: Why do you think it felt good?

ADOLESCENT: Because we were together, just the two of us.

THERAPIST: A mother and her young boy.

ADOLESCENT: Yeah.

THERAPIST: And that was the only moment you remember being close to her?

ADOLESCENT: That's it.

THERAPIST: That sounds like an important memory to you.

ADOLESCENT: I guess so.

THERAPIST: But maybe sad too, because you realize that you were alone so much of your childhood – a time when parents are taking closer care of their children.

ADOLESCENT: She was okay.

THERAPIST: I know. It just sounds as if she was unable to take proper care of you.

ADOLESCENT: She didn't have to. I could do it myself.

THERAPIST: So she expected something unrealistic from you, and you rose to the challenge?

ADOLESCENT: What do you mean?

THERAPIST: Well, most parents don't expect their 7-year-old sons to fend for themselves.

ADOLESCENT: I know some people who do that to their kids.

THERAPIST: Yeah, so do I. But that's too bad. Most kids need their parents to be around – show them the way, protect them, take care of them.

ADOLESCENT: Do we have to keep talking about this? It's boring.

THERAPIST: I think it's boring and maybe also a little uncomfortable for you, because it brings up sad or mad feelings. Just one last thing, and we'll get off this subject. Do you see any relationship between your feeling like you had to take care of your-self as a child, and the fact that you are feeling angry at your foster parents about trying to watch you too much?

ADOLESCENT: Well, first of all, it's too late for that. I grew up already. Secondly, they are not my parents, and I don't think they should be treating me like I was their kid. I'm not. I have my real mother, even though she doesn't care about me.

THERAPIST: Okay, so we'll stop talking about this now, but I think you've made a good beginning. I think there is a relationship between what happened to you as a child and what is happening to you now, and it has something to do with thoughts and feelings you've kept to yourself for years.

Eventually, this boy was able to see that he had defended himself against tremendous loneliness and fear by developing a facade of toughness: As long as he didn't care whether his mother showed up or not, he avoided disappointment. He took care of himself by needing no one, and he was now terrified of trusting the foster parents (who, by the way, had offered to adopt him) or allowing himself to depend on them for anything. As long as he was self-sufficient, he was safe. This process of connecting the dots allowed him to understand that there was a way in which he was responding to his mother as he interacted with his foster parents, and a way in which these responses interfered with the possibility of his building new and rewarding interpersonal relationships. We continued to work on past issues only as they were found to be obstacles to current functioning.

I think it's also worth noting that some youngsters overemphasize the significance of past events on current functioning. Ralph, for example, a 15-year-old youth who is best described as a "class scapegoat," was always being teased and beaten-up in school. Although he never precipitated arguments with school friends, he was constantly involved in altercations. When we met, I asked him why he thought he was always getting hurt by classmates at school.

"I don't know why. Kids just don't like me. They're always calling me names, and I don't know how to fight back." I continued to explore his perceptions of his predicament and finally, in a resigned manner, he said, "I've been getting beaten all my life. My dad used to beat me all the time when I was a kid. When he died I figured it would stop, but no, now it's just other people who do it. I guess I just bring out the worst in people."

There was something in this youngster's mannerisms that elicited strong countertransference responses in me: It was difficult for me to empathize with him, I felt frustrated and annoyed, and I even experienced wanting to reject him (i.e., refer him to another therapist). Once I processed my reactions I realized that this youngster presented himself as a helpless victim whose fate was sealed. He epitomized the concept "learned helplessness," and he had learned to see his life through a single lens: He was an abused child and he would always be abused by someone.

I worked with Ralph for about 9 months, and contrary to my initial expectations, he was one of the most rewarding cases I ever saw. We did some specific work on his self-view, view of others as more powerful than himself, and restricted view of interactions as including a victim and a victimizer. He responded very well to group therapy, and finally developed relationships with peers that did not entail violence and humiliation. As others regarded him more positively, his self-concept changed as well. There was a dramatic change in his physical posture and his pitch and tone of voice. Ralph agreed that although his past had included violence and pain, it was possible to establish rewarding and safe interactions with others.

I did focus a portion of the therapy on Ralph's prior abuse and Ralph was able to have a cathartic release which he found very helpful. In all the years he had been beaten, Ralph had never cried (or made any sounds) because Ralph learned early on that his father would beat him more when he did. In one of our sessions Ralph wept openly, and grieved for the childhood he had not had. This session, more than any other, allowed Ralph to become more emotionally available to myself, the therapy process, and presumably to others.

Finding Alternative Responses

Although challenging established belief systems, ascertaining their origins, and gaining new understanding and insight are important steps in the process of disengaging from the past and feeling more in control of current functioning, insight is not sufficient to cause change. Once the dots are connected and the relationship between past and present is made explicit, the next challenge is that of finding healthier coping strategies and using defensive strategies only when these are realistically needed. Abused adolescents seem to have reflex responses to certain situations, based on their prior experiences. When youngsters have had painful experiences with women, for example, their expectations may be that all women will be hurtful or uncaring. Consequently, such a youngster may see a female therapist, and his or her guard goes up. This is an automatic, generalized response, often without conscious awareness – not unlike the reaction of certain animals that expel noxious or venomous fluids when they sense danger.

What I encourage adolescents to do is to begin to monitor their own feelings and their physical and emotional responses. They might begin by recognizing that they feel "uncomfortable" or "funny," when they are alone in a room with an adult, or when they have to interact with an older or younger person. Then, once the acknowledgment is made, they explore their reactions, amplifying their awareness of how their bodies react and what kinds of feelings get generated. Tolerating these uncomfortable feelings is an important strategy for change through self-control: If youngsters can recognize that certain things are happening to them, they can then "sit with" the feelings and watch what happens.

I make the process of affect tolerance a type of game that adolescents can view as a challenge. I say something like this:

> "When you feel that uncomfortable feeling, and you've pinpointed lots of helpful information about how you know you're in an uncomfortable situation, I want you to 'stand your feelings' as long as you can. And I'm sure as time goes by, you'll be able to tolerate these feelings and sensations for longer and longer

periods of time. For now, I will set a timer for 30 seconds, and when the bell rings we can talk together and you won't need to feel your feelings any more. Obviously, with kids who have done this successfully for a period of time, I set the timer for longer. But since you're new at this and not so experienced, we'll set it for a little bit shorter time."

I set the timer for a short span, and then challenge them to go beyond the initial bell. Youngsters in group therapy often compete with their more experienced counterparts, going well beyond the initial period of affect tolerance. This tangible way of helping children expand their abilities to tolerate their affect is usually very beneficial. Youngsters need to know that they will not die from feeling their feelings, they will not overwhelm others, and they will be able to tolerate their feelings – all contrary to what they may suspect.

Once young clients become proficient at this skill, we begin to talk about what they can do instead of squelching the feelings they have. Usually this involves acknowledgment, acceptance, honoring, processing, and coping or self-soothing in a healthy manner. Although these steps sound reasonable and facile, they are difficult steps to take and maintain.

Acknowledgment, the first step, means that youngsters recognize and acknowledge to themselves or others that something is troubling them. I always give youngsters the choice of telling or not telling about something they have just acknowledged to themselves. Some adolescents prefer to discuss issues privately in individual therapy, or may choose to raise them instead in the safety of a group setting.

Acceptance of feelings implies that youngsters allow themselves to have a feeling without judging it. So often adolescents (and adults) evaluate their feelings according to whether they "should" or "should not" have them, or whether they think they are "right" or "wrong." As long as feelings are appraised in this way, it is more difficult for an individual to say, "I have this feeling right now. I'm not sure why it's here, or what happened to bring it on, but I feel really weird, and I want to explore it some more."

I then instruct youngsters to honor their feelings by saying to themselves (or others), "I honor my feelings by letting them be, by not trying to make them right or wrong, and by knowing that they are there for good reasons. There is a lesson to be learned from this particular feeling's presence at this time."

Processing means an active exploration of feelings, with attempts to trace their origins (predisposing factors), triggers (precipitating factors), and forces that might keep the problem current (perpetuating factors).

The last step, coping or self-soothing, assumes individuals' innate ability to cope with difficult emotions in a healthy manner, and to draw upon inner resources to comfort and reconstitute themselves.

The following example, reconstructed from my memory of a group therapy session, as well as from sketchy clinical notes, illustrates how I encourage youngsters to tolerate and work through uncomfortable emotions. The young clients in this group had been in therapy for over a year, so they were familiar with the concepts outlined above, and were cooperating very well with one another and with the group leaders. Observe how a relatively innocuous issue elicited strong emotions that were processed in the group:

THERAPIST 1: Okay, okay, guys, I think we need to move on. I think you all did a good job of catching up with each other after our break, and it's time to get started.

THERAPIST 2: Who remembers what we talked about in our last group?

CLIENT 1: I know, I know, it was about that boundary thing and how we're supposed to respect each other's space.

THERAPIST 1: Good, that's right. We talked about boundaries. Who remembers more?

CLIENT 2: Wait, wait. Before we start, I need to tell S. that he gots a cool haircut.

THERAPIST 1: Okay, now remember, that's the kind of comment we do during snack time. We've moved on now to the group discussion.

CLIENT 2: I know, I know, I just forgot to tell him, that's all.

CLIENT 4: Thanks, dude.

THERAPIST 1: Okay, now what else do you remember about what was discussed last time?

[This discussion goes on for another 10 minutes.]

CLIENT 5: I think there's something wrong with B [Client 3].

THERAPIST 2: Ask B. directly if you think there's something wrong.

CLIENT 5: Is there something wrong with you?

CLIENT 3: No, man, leave me alone. (*Obviously disgruntled and uncharacteristically withdrawn*)

THERAPIST 2: You've been very quiet, B. Take a minute and see if you can let us know what's going on inside you.

[We wait about 5 minutes, and B. cries.]

THERAPIST 1: Obviously, something is troubling you right now.

CLIENT 3: I just feel weird, that's what.

THERAPIST 2: Okay, you feel weird. Say some more about feeling weird.

CLIENT 3: My feelings . . . they got hurt.

THERAPIST 2: Your feelings got hurt. Did that happen in the group or before you got to group?

CLIENT 3: During the group.

THERAPIST 2: Okay, you're doing a good job acknowledging that something's wrong. That's the first step. And whatever it is, it happened here in the group.

CLIENT 3: Okay.

CLIENT 6: Maybe he didn't remember about last week and he felt bad.

THERAPIST 1: That's a good guess. Check it out.

CLIENT 6: Is that it, B.?

CLIENT 3: Nah.

THERAPIST 2: If you can, tell us when you first noticed your feelings getting hurt.

CLIENT 3: (*After a long pause*) When he told S. that his haircut was cool.

CLIENT 2: Huh? How come you tripped on that?

CLIENT 3: See . . . I don't want no problems with you, man.

THERAPIST 2: Okay, for now, I want you to stay focused on yourself. We'll talk to [Client 2] later. Do you know what it was about S. complimenting M.'s haircut that hurt your feelings?

CLIENT 3: It just reminded me, that's all.

THERAPIST 2: Reminded you of what?

CLIENT 3: Of all the times people have tripped on my hair and ragged on me about it.

THERAPIST 1: Who tripped on your hair?

CLIENT 3: My dad, my mom, my brother, my teachers, my friends.

THERAPIST 1: Wow, that's a lot of people. How come?

CLIENT 3: 'Cause my hair was really, really curly, and it didn't look like anybody else's in my family.

THERAPIST 1: I don't notice that your hair is particularly curly.

CLIENT 3: That's 'cause I blow-dry it and put mousse on it.

THERAPIST 1: So you take great care to make sure your hair looks the way you want it.

CLIENT 3: Yeah.

THERAPIST 2: And do kids still rag on you?

CLIENT 3: No, not really . . . but I always think they will.

THERAPIST 2: So back to the comment about M. How did you hear that?

CLIENT 3: This is gonna sound crazy, but when S. said he liked M.'s hair, all I heard was that he didn't like mine.

CLIENT 2: I never said that!

THERAPIST 1: I think he knows you never said that. He's just saying that that's what he heard because he's sensitive to hair comments.

CLIENT 3: Whenever anybody brings up hair, I don't like it. I freak, man.

THERAPIST 1: And when you freak, what does that feel like?

CLIENT 3: I just get quiet and my feelings hurt.

THERAPIST 1: How do you feel, mostly?

CLIENT 3: I don't know. Sad, I guess.

THERAPIST 1: And what do you do with the sad feeling?

CLIENT 3: I try to tell myself not to feel it, 'cause it's stupid, and 'cause nobody did nothing to me.

THERAPIST 1: And when you try to stop your feelings, does it work?

CLIENT 3: Not always. Sometimes.

THERAPIST 2: When does it work?

CLIENT 3: When I forget about it by doing something else.

THERAPIST 2: Any other time?

CLIENT 3: Sometimes . . .

THERAPIST 2: And what happens if you let yourself feel the feeling for a while?

CLIENT 3: I get more sad.

THERAPIST 2: Is that all?

CLIENT 3: Well, I get quiet.

THERAPIST 2: And what happens when you are quiet?

CLIENT 3: Well, not here, but other places the kids forget about me.

THERAPIST 1: What do you mean?

CLIENT 3: They don't notice me after a while.

THERAPIST 1: And how does that feel?

CLIENT 3: Not good.

THERAPIST 1: How?

CLIENT 3: Kind of bad.

THERAPIST 1: Okay, so what else can you do rather than getting quiet when you have an uncomfortable feeling?

CLIENT 3: I know, I know, talk about it.

THERAPIST 2: Now how would that help?

CLIENT 3: You know.

THERAPIST 2: I just wanna make sure you know.

CLIENT 3: Well, when I talk, I can figure things out better, and I stay part of the group.

THERAPIST 2: That's terrific. That's exactly why it helps to talk. How are you feeling now?

CLIENT 3: Okay, mostly.

THERAPIST 2: Still sad?

CLIENT 3: Not as much. Some.

THERAPIST 2: And how do others feel?

CLIENT 5: My mom makes fun of my freckles and I hate it. I'm always waiting for somebody to say something about them.

THERAPIST 1: And how do you feel when somebody says something about your freckles?

CLIENT 5: Bad.

THERAPIST 2: Anybody else got something they feel sensitive about?

[The discussion continues. Finally, Therapist 1 summarizes the session in the following manner:]

THERAPIST 1: And I want to thank S. for noticing that something was wrong with B. and for asking him. What B. shared with us today was relevant to everyone in the group. That is, there are times when we feel sensitive about something (like hair, freckles, weight, or other things), and because we are sensitive we can read into comments that are made. Like when S. compliment-ed M. on his haircut, B. thought that was a putdown of him, because no comment was made about his hair. He read a criti-cism into S.'s compliment to M., because he expects that peo-ple are going to criticize him about his hair. It's like when someone says, "You look good today," and you say, "What do you mean, *today*?" At face value that's a compliment, but on the receiving end you're making it something else. Right? I also want to thank B. for choosing to talk about his feelings out loud and becoming a part of the group.

In this group session, therefore, B. acknowledged his vulnera-bility to comments about hair; he remembered being teased about his hair from the time he was very young (the predisposing factor); he reacted to a positive comment that one group member made about another group member's hair (the precipitating factor); and, although he initially became sullen and withdrawn (perpetuating factor), he was able to respond well to a group member's attention and chose to trust the group with his difficult emotions, thereby breaking the response that perpetuated negative feelings. B. was able to ac-knowledge and honor his feelings, as well as process them, so that he could advance toward healthier goals: remaining part of the group rather than withdrawing, and expressing himself rather than retreat-ing and wallowing in unpleasant thoughts and feelings.

Addressing the Facts and Impact of Abuse

Acknowledgment of the type, extent, and impact of childhood abuse is one of the earliest steps that abused adolescents must take in ord-er to put the past behind them and exercise more control over their lives. Many adolescents don't like to rehash their past experiences; others talk about them incessantly, emphasizing their victimization and appearing victim-like in their current lives, even when the abuse has long since ceased.

When adolescents are resistant to talking about their pasts, I agree with them that the goal is to move on. The question, then, is "How do we help abused individuals move on?" Clearly, there is no single way that helps everyone, but there are some basic steps that facilitate moving on – especially acknowledgment and process- ing. Abused individuals need to achieve clarity about what happened to them, develop a realistic view of how those early events may or may not have repercussions in aspects of their current function- ing, and achieve closure. In other words, youngsters must confront either their denial of facts, or their fixation on events that cannot be relived. I often tell adolescents, "You cannot go back and relive what happened to you as a child. What you do have control over is what happens to you from this point forward." Just as individu- als may develop various types of denial, such as rationalization, minimization, and partial admission, acknowledgment also may be fractional or incomplete and may remain so for short or long peri- ods of time. Often denial is challenged by other events, such as a child abuse report from a younger sibling, a police investigation, or other legal involvement, as well as through the process of maturation.

There are many reasons why adolescents deny abuse. Loyalty appears to be one of the most common reasons: Adolescents may feel that if they "tell," they are badmouthing their parents. Converse- ly, youngsters who can only find fault with their parents may be stuck in making their disappointment known to others in an effort to stay safe, get help, or get even.

Dealing with Issues of Denial

It's important to recognize that denial does not occur in a vacuum; adolescents often find it necessary to protect themselves against pain- ful truths. I tend to accept and expect denial in adolescent clients early in treatment. I assume that if I become trustworthy enough, or create a safe enough setting, denial will decrease or subside al- together.

I find it absolutely counterproductive to engage in power strug- gles with adolescents (or others) regarding "facts" early in treatment. Realistically, therapeutic trust usually precedes full admission of per- sonal or painful information.

If I'm working with adolescents who are referred because they have committed a crime (such as a sexual offense), I always obtain a copy of the police or probation report; I simply read the facts to the adolescent, asserting that these are facts we will need to discuss at some later time, although I don't expect them to feel comfortable doing so at this point in treatment. As a matter of fact, when I worked at A Step Forward in Concord, California, my colleague Jeff Bodmer-Turner (who specializes in the treatment of adolescents and adults who have committed sexual offenses) and I would meet with families of adolescents, and tell the adolescents that their job initially was to listen to everyone's concerns and reactions. They would not be required to make any statements until later in treatment.

Another idea that has served me well is to allow peers, rather than authority figures (e.g., probation officers, social workers, or therapists), to confront denial. I have facilitated many group meetings with new members in denial, in which the task of the group has been to discuss the many ways in which denial is useful. It appears to be helpful to make explicit that denial serves as a necessary psychological defense in the short run, and that acknowledging the truth and asking for help will have positive consequences in the long run.

When Should Trauma Be Processed?

With resistant youths, or with youngsters who speak dispassionately and continually about the abuse, I may emphasize different things. Although these two types of youths appear quite different at first glance, they are mostly cut from the same cloth. The child who vehemently refuses to discuss the past, or who denies either the facts or their impact, may be trying to defend against painful feelings. Likewise, the youngster who talks incessantly and provides explicit details without affect – that is, as if the abuse happened to someone else – may also be protecting against painful feelings. As long as this second youth keeps talking to different people, and providing often shocking facts regarding his or her abuse, no true processing occurs. Both youngsters remain preoccupied with issues of past abuse, and this preoccupation probably interferes with functioning in some small or large way. At a minimum, rigorous self-disclosure may keep people at arm's length; again, this may be viewed as safer than actually trusting people, getting feedback, or moving beyond the reporting of facts.

Often, abused adolescents have been traumatized by their experiences; as previously discussed, they may develop symptoms of PTSD (e.g., intrusive thoughts and flashbacks, auditory hallucinations, physical sensations, emotional outbursts [or, conversely, numbing], and nightmares in which the original trauma material appears). These symptoms may be triggered by a range of environmental stimuli, and an adolescent may defend against the symptoms by dissociating, particularly if his or her primary defense at the time of the trauma was dissociation.

The issue of directly addressing past abuse in therapy elicits heated debate among mental health professionals, and rightfully so. In my experience, the question of whether or not the abuse material should be addressed directly must be answered by the client himself or herself and by the nature of the presenting problem. I believe that abuse will probably need to be processed directly in a structured way when the following conditions exist:

1. Acute or chronic PTSD symptoms.
2. Worrisome symptomatic behaviors (e.g., self-injury, substance abuse, suicidal ideation, aggressive sexual acting out), and/or a social history of a chaotic, violent, or neglectful background.
3. Chronic reenactments of abuse dynamics (e.g., revictimizations, offending behavior, learned helplessness).
4. Vigorous denial of any history of abuse, or of the impact of those experiences; or indiscriminate, affect-free disclosures of victimization.

When traumatic material is addressed and processed, this must be done in a safe environment in which the therapist helps the client to acknowledge, honor, and work through difficult thoughts, feelings, and questions, and guides the process with a focus on the goals of integration and self-control. Clinicians will have varied ways to accomplish these goals, and extraordinary care must be taken to pursue these issues only with adolescents who have learned an array of coping strategies, have a fortified sense of self, and have reinforced their internal resources so that they can create safety for themselves. Herman (1992) cautions that the single most frequent therapeutic error is failing to address the patient's traumatic material, and the next most frequent clinical error is premature, or overzealous pursuit of traumatic material. Chapter Five provides a detailed description of the structured processing of trauma.

Cognitive Reassessments: Shifting Perceptions

One of the areas requiring constant attention is that of cognitive reassessment, particularly as developmental maturation takes place, or new experiences provide data that support or contradict prior perceptions. Cognitive reassessments can be either positive or negative. For example, one young adult woman was raped by a man who was captured, tried, and convicted. During the trial, other women testified to being raped; this young woman was shocked to learn that the other victims had been raped at gunpoint, and that the police suspected this rapist of having killed yet another of his victims. Once she acknowledged how close to death she had been during the rape, particularly in light of the fact that her rapist was suspected of actual murder, she had a relapse in which acute PTSD symptoms resurfaced and debilitated her for 3–4 months. In this case, her cognitive reassessment had a negative impact, in that she felt worse – more vulnerable, more anxious – after she realized the grave danger she had escaped.

Conversely, a 49-year-old woman was relieved and empowered once she reevaluated her childhood abuse with full adult cognitive capacity. She had always believed that she had caused the abuse because she had not been able to say "no," choosing instead to pretend to be asleep. Once we discussed how falling asleep was a way of saying "no," she stopped blaming herself and shifted responsibility to the man who had molested her. "After all," she asked rhetorically, "what kind of man takes advantage of a little girl who's asleep?" This reevaluation allowed her to view herself, and her attempts to stop the abuse, in a new and more positive way.

Expanding Self-Image and Positive Identity

As the second example just above suggests, new input about earlier experiences and why they occurred may allow adolescents to view themselves in a more positive light. Andy, a 15-year-old boy abandoned by his parents when he was quite young, had always harbored a belief that there was something inherently wrong with him: "Why else would my folks split on me? I must have been a real piece of work!" This youngster needed a lot of evidence to counter this belief system (which protected his parents' image while it sacrificed his own).

Andy had been 4 years old when his parents disappeared, leaving him and his younger sister in a motel room. One of my therapeutic interventions directed him to spend time around 4-year-olds. He had a friend with a young brother and offered to babysit with his friend a few times. After "hanging out" with his friend and his brother, Andy reported that the 4-year-old was "cool, liked to play, and was easy to get along with." He was struck by how small his friend's brother was, and wondered whether he himself had been that small (he had no photographs of himself as a child, which often made him wonder how he had looked). I also asked Andy to try to spend some time with the child when his friends' parents were around. After doing so, he stated, "They were cool with him. The dad yelled once but then he was cool, and the kid was really glad to see the dad when he got home, and the mom made him eat the food on his plate but she gave him small amounts." I asked whether the child had been "bad," and, if so, what his parents had done when he was bad. Andy looked up at me with surprise in his face, saying, "He's not bad, he's just a kid, and when he did something wrong his parents just told him to chill out." This was a very powerful, concrete lesson for Andy, who realized that children were not inherently bad. They were, however, inherently dependent, eager to please, and loving toward their parents.

Andy and I then discussed the circumstances precipitating his entry into the foster care system. I asked his social worker to track down records about the youngster's placement, and she retrieved important information: Andy's parents had been "in the system" for years. My client and his younger sister were only two of five children who had been removed from the mother and father's care. The parents were drug addicts who often engaged in illegal activities to get money to buy drugs. They had been arrested a few times for fraud and for passing bad checks. The social worker who conducted the evaluation and filed for termination of parental rights noted that the parents viewed having children as a way of establishing an income without working. The previous three children had been removed for gross neglect and physical abuse; they had been adopted separately.

Andy's social worker, his foster (later adoptive) parents, and I met to discuss how much of this information would be useful for Andy to know. Because of his persistently negative self-image, and the fact that he conserved an idealized vision of his parents (at his own expense), we decided to give him all the facts we could, including the fact that his three older siblings had also been taken away and placed for adoption. We spent considerable time making this decision and discussing whether Andy's knowledge of the older siblings' existence might cause him more distress. Our decision was that there was a greater advantage to his knowing the truth, in that it might help him view himself more objectively – not as a child who was bad, but a child whom his parents could not care for, just as they hadn't been able to care for the others.

As his therapist, I was assigned the task of relaying this information about his childhood to Andy. He was intensely interested in whatever minimal information there was about his parents, who had long since been "unknown" to the system. His foster parents had always felt that they would support Andy's efforts to locate his parents once he turned 18; Andy had known his parents' names since he was very young.

Andy asked whether I was sure that his parents had three older children, and asked what their names and ages were. I gave him whatever sketchy information was available, and he seemed very interested to hear that his siblings would now be in their 20s, although there was no information on their adoptive parents. He sat quiet for a while after hearing the full story for the first time.

"So they just couldn't handle having little kids around," was his first comment. "Some people simply aren't cut out to be parents," I responded. He went on: "Wow, what a racket, trying to get paid for having kids." "Unfortunately," I told him, "I've run into that kind of welfare scam a couple of times."

Over the next few months there was a dramatic change in Andy. His realization that his parents had abandoned not only him and his sister, but three of his older siblings as well, allowed him to see himself differently. "I wonder if I was like my buddy's brother," he said at one of our meetings. "What do you think?" I asked. He replied, "Well, probably, because we like the same kind of things, and he even looks a little like me . . . maybe I would have looked like that when I was little." Andy had identified with his friend's brother and was reevaluating his views about children, their inherent goodness, and the fact that some individuals actually enjoy being parents and do their jobs well.

Believing that there was nothing inherently bad, unlovable, or unworthy about himself gave Andy a new perspective on his strengths and positive characteristics. He began to excel academically, and his acting-out behaviors declined. He also became more emotionally available, not only in the therapy sessions, but with his friends and foster family as well. Eventually, Andy and his sister were formally adopted by his foster parents, and it was as if he and the parents had chosen each other. "I finally feel like I belong to somebody, like somebody really wants me," he said, "no matter how jerky I act sometimes."

Developing an Orientation toward Personal Safety

Andy, the youngster in the preceding example, was a "good kid" who struggled with his negative self-image. As a result, he often made poor choices and used poor judgment about whom to befriend. He had originally been referred to treatment because of joy-riding. His academic performance had always been adequate, but his behavior at school was sporadically problematic.

After the therapy interventions mentioned above, I began working with Andy on acting on his own behalf instead of sabotaging himself. "Now that you've figured out that you were born a good kid, always were a good kid, and continue to be a good kid, you need to make decisions that support that point of view." We reframed this attention to himself as a way to keep himself safe and not put himself in harm's way: "Now that you're getting older, it's your turn to make decisions for yourself. Experiment with making sure you know what your options are, and which of the options supports your new view of yourself as opposed to your old view of yourself." Andy agreed to this and became excited about finding opportunities to make good choices.

One clear example was choosing to approach his foster parents and broach the subject of adoption. His foster parents had brought the topic up for years, but Andy had always refused. Although he felt he took an emotional risk in talking to them about adoption, he acted on his own behalf, asserting his right to be part of a family that he had grown to love, and that had loved him and his sister for years.

Andy also made better personal choices about friends. In spite of the fact that his old friends persisted in calling him and coming by his house, he set firm limits on his homework time, often forgoing or delaying social activities until he was done.

Andy told me that he often said to himself, "You've got to do this for you, man. You've got to give yourself a leg up." His new positive self-image motivated his behavior and allowed him to feel optimistic about his future.

Beyond Trauma Processing:
Empowerment, Affiliation, Future Orientation

In the last several years I have been interested in, and influenced by, narrative therapy. This approach regards the individual as capable of making change, and provides a focus for learning based on what the individual already knows (from experience) about how to solve a problem. Narrative therapy concerns itself mostly with how the person creates a story about who he or she is (i.e., the person's sense of self) and what his or her life has been like so far. In particular, narrative therapists believe that when an individual creates a story, he or she may over time become exclusively committed to the story, which then becomes a foundation for the development of attitudes, beliefs, and behaviors. Because of the obvious implications for abused children, who often develop a negative sense of self as a result of prior experiences, or who may have been affected by the powerful lessons of abuse that influence expectations and perceptions, a narrative approach can be very helpful for abused adolescents.

Andy, for example, created a narrative that began with a limited perception of the events that had occurred in his life. As a 4-year-old who had been abandoned by his parents, he told himself (and others) that something intrinsically defective about him had caused his parents to turn away from him. This belief influenced how he interacted with others (not trusting them, not allowing himself to get close, and then emphasizing others' rejection), as well as the kinds of situations he approached or withdrew from (since he felt basically inadequate, he didn't risk failure and withdrew from competition or academic endeavors).

In therapy Andy rescripted his personal narrative, including new information about his parents, their accountability in having children they were not willing or able to care for, and their pattern of bringing children into the world without first creating a safe and nurturing environment. His new narrative was that he had been a "good kid," loving and willing to please, and that his parents had not had the maturity or ability to build responsible lives for themselves. Finally, Andy projected a story about his future and imagined himself as a capable, caring, responsible adult who would create a family different from that of his biological parents. He had grown to see himself as someone with a lot to offer to children and peers. During his senior year in high school, he became a successful peer counselor and began talking about wanting to prepare for a job as a counselor with troubled youths.

A narrative approach seeks to create a balanced self-view, rather than one dominated by one perspective. Durrant and Kowalski (1990), extrapolating from White and Epston's (1990) guiding principles, note their concern with a recent trend in the United States: Some adult survivors of childhood abuse are developing an "abuse-dominated view" of themselves, or building their identities exclusively around their experience of victimization. Certainly it appears that the narrative of victimization, particularly when a modicum of safety has been created, can affect a person's sense of safety, vulnerability, optimism, and/or willingness to engage in specific behaviors and not others.

The narrative approach redirects and expands an individual's focus to information that he or she may have previously overlooked or minimized. For example, if a boy talks about his "drunk father who never had time for me," questioning might focus on times the father was not drunk, times the father did make time for the youngster, or any other information challenging the view that the boy's father was "always" drunk and unavailable. Even if the adolescent cannot come up with alternative information, questions might focus on who else did have time for him, and who else in his life never had a drinking problem.

The narrative approach is particularly helpful with adolescents who believe that they have been vulnerable or helpless in their lives. Helping them recognize how they took care of themselves when they were in danger, or how they tried to stop the abuse, can change these youths' self-view. For example, Anna was 15 years old and had a substance abuse problem. When she was sober, she was plagued with feelings of despair. Often she would say, "Life isn't what it's cracked up to be. Sometimes I wish it would stop now." I frequently responded, "Your life hasn't been easy so far, and I know you want the pain to stop. That's why you drink, it seems, so you don't feel the hurt." "What do I do?" she would plead, and I would say the one thing she didn't want to hear: "You've got to let yourself feel your feelings, and we've got to talk about what did happen to you and why." "I know why," she retorted. "I'm just plain no good."

Working with Anna was a challenge, in that she had developed such a strong belief that she had been hurt because she was unworthy of love. She also felt responsible for being sexually abused by her father, believing that she had "led him on" by being orgasmic during the sexual abuse. Many youngsters have difficulty with their bodies' responding with pleasure to the abuse. They believe that if they had physical sensations, this means they were responsible for the fact that the sexual abuse happened. They feel like co-conspirators, and guilt prevails. For Anna, it was important for her to realize that she loved her father and longed for his attention and affection. However, she did not ask for, nor did she have control over, the sexual abuse.

As we explored some of Anna's feelings, she stumbled over the fact that she mostly felt bad because she had not said the word "No." When I asked her if she had ever said "No" nonverbally, she remembered that shortly after she was first sexually abused, she had put a safety pin at the top of a zipper on her sleeper pajamas. She seemed excited by the notion that she had said "No" nonverbally, but disappointed by the fact that she had not been successful in stopping the abuse. Finally, when I asked her to think about how she had said "Yes," she sat up and asserted, "I never told him he could do it!" Finally she began to realize that her father did not concern himself with whether or not she said "Yes" or "No." He was sexually abusing her because he could, because he had control, and because she was vulnerable and loving.

Anna still had difficulty reconciling her orgasmic behavior with her lack of responsibility for the abuse; somehow, she viewed this as "proof" that she was just as bad as her "pervert father." I did a very concrete (and symbolic) intervention with Anna—one that I had tried on much younger children before. I brought a red onion into the office, and much to her amazement I cut it. Shortly thereafter, we both cried.

"What's happening?" I asked Anna. "We're bawling," she responded.

"What do you make of that?" I asked her, and she quickly answered, "It's the onion smell."

"Yep," I added. "I'm not sad, you're not sad, and there's nothing to cry about. And yet, when our noses smell the onion, our eyes leak tears. I think there's a lesson to be learned from this."

I put the onion away, asked Anna to think about what had just happened, and went to wash my hands. When I returned she had a smile in her face and a tear in her eye. I sat down and heard words that were music to my ears: "It's like what happened to my body . . . when he touched me in certain places, I got wet, and I got off." She now had a way of understanding that her orgasm was not compliance with sexual abuse, but a way in which her body reacted to sexual stimulation. Anna now had a new narrative about her early experiences.

CONCLUSIONS

The goals of treatment with previously abused adolescents range from addressing generic issues such as identity, self-esteem, autonomy, family conflicts, feelings of isolation, values clarification, sexuality, peer pressure, and specific presenting complaints (substance abuse, depression, suicidality, eating disorders) to addressing issues generally associated with abuse: guilt, shame, sexual identity problems, youth prostitution and running away (Burgess & Hartman, 1995), feelings of betrayal or helplessness, anger, relationship difficulties, and reliance on psychological defenses such as denial or dissociation.

Adolescents are usually referred for therapy because their behavior is a problem or concern to someone else. Although they may not initially be "voluntary clients," my experience is that adolescents eventually come to value the opportunity to be heard and understood, and appreciate having someone they may perceive to be an advocate or ally. Karen (1994) notes: " . . . it would seem important to reach insecurely attached children by adolescence, because that's when it's believed their patterns become more firmly set. Even then they can still be changed; there is still the possibility of psychotherapy, not to mention other vital relationships, and the emotional flux of the adolescent years sometimes opens children up in new ways" (p. 232).

Many abused adolescents do not see how past abuse relates to current problems. Others however, have learned to use past abuse as an explanation for every problem they face. Yet other adolescents seem to reenact abuse dynamics, exhibiting either identification with aggressors, or experiences of victimization. It is imperative to make careful assessments to determine the most helpful interventions for adolescents with histories of abuse. The overriding goal, however, is to improve the youngster's overall functioning, remove obstacles to ongoing development, and assist with the development of personal power, safety, and mastery.

How these goals are addressed will differ from clinician to clinician, and until we conduct treatment outcome studies to help us determine which specific techniques seem to help the most (or the most quickly), we will need to use good theory coupled with good ethics to inform and shape our treatment interventions. In addition, we must make ongoing efforts to develop treatment plans with measurable goals, incorporate self-report instruments to gauge changes in the client's mood or behavior, and develop standardized methods of accountability including peer review, consultation, and client satisfaction reports. I have long used a practice of having clients evaluate the treatment (both in person and in writing) during termination and I use this feedback as one measure of my contribution to clients' improved functioning.

As noted earlier, the question of whether or not to address past abuse directly in therapy has been a controversial topic among clinicians, and justifiably so. My experience suggests that this question should be answered by the individual client and by the nature of his or her presenting problem. I believe that abuse will generally need to be addressed directly in a structured manner under the conditions described earlier in this chapter. In these cases, adolescents will need a safe environment in which to acknowledge, honor, and process their thoughts and feelings, as well as guidance in altering problem behaviors so that they are functioning in their own best interests.

Therapists will have varied methods of accomplishing these goals, and extraordinary care must be taken to pursue these issues with adolescents who have a strengthened sense of self, an array of internal resources and coping strategies, and feelings of safety. Techniques such as regressive therapies, hypnosis for purposes of accessing memories, the use of intrusive psychopharmacological measures (e.g., amobarbital), and dream work to resolve abuse issues have not been proven necessary, and have disadvantages that cannot be overlooked. In the next chapter, I discuss techniques for processing trauma that I have found useful.

CHAPTER FIVE

Structured Processing of Trauma

Individuals who were abused as children have differing responses to their experiences, depending on a number of variables – not the least of which are the chronicity and severity of the abuse. When the abuse is not chronic or severe, and when survivors get adequate protection after abusive incidents, recovery may occur more quickly. Some survivors are able to acknowledge the event and its impact more readily, give the experiences accurate meaning, place the responsibility on the abusers, view the events as unusual (and as such don't expect them to be repeated), get adequate nurturing and support from their family and/or friends, and seem able to move on without feeling overwhelmed or permanently debilitated. These individuals may be called "resilient," or may be responding to the reparative qualities of an appropriate and safe environment. Moreover, when the abuse is acute, it's precipitants may be resolved quickly. On occasion I have worked with abusive individuals who confide that the very first act of child abuse served as an antidote to further abuse, such was their shock at having lost control of their emotions and behavior.

Sometimes when abuse is severe, protective agencies become involved, and in some cases children are removed from their homes temporarily or permanently. Several clients have mentioned the relief they felt when they went into foster care; they also knew that they had recourse if their parents or other caretakers should injure them again. Many other survivors are not as fortunate and relate stories of chronic or severe abuse that has long-term consequences.

Often long-term consequences are either minimized by, or exacerbated by, experiences that occur after the abuse itself. Jonathan and Wayne were both 15-year-old adolescents who had been removed from their homes at age 13 following severe physical abuse from stepparents. Jonathan went into a group home; his mother and stepfather received family counseling; and he was able to continue to attend school without the disruption of transfer. After 6 months he was returned to his family, and the abuse did not recur. Wayne was not as fortunate: He was physically abused in his group home by a staff member; his parents did not receive counseling and had subsequent marital problems; and he remained in foster care for 2 years, in a total of six placements. Wayne related to adults with great defensiveness and mistrust, expecting to be assaulted or criticized. Jonathan was far more receptive to positive efforts from others. In Jonathan's case, what occurred after his abuse was helpful and restored his family's functioning. In Wayne's case, the interventions designed to be helpful probably exacerbated the impact of the original abuse.

As I have stated in Chapter Four, I believe that abuse issues must be confronted in a direct, structured way in some, but not all, cases. Careful assessments must uncover the extent of the individual's involvement with abuse-related material—that is, how much of his or her current difficulty in functioning can be directly traced to unresolved issues with the abuse. In my experience, the individuals who have been traumatized by abuse experiences and who have failed to process the traumatic material are the ones who most urgently require an in-depth exploration, processing, and closure of their past experiences.

Simply put, processing trauma involves acknowledging the facts of abuse and their impact; experiencing and releasing some of the feelings associated with the trauma that may have been left unexpressed; exploring a range of feelings toward victimizers and nonprotective parents, siblings, or caretakers; and making cognitive reassessments of the abuse (i.e., why it happened, who was responsible, etc.). If these avenues are explored, the traumatic event is faced and activated by necessity; it can no longer remain "frozen in time," maintaining its status quo. The status quo may include beliefs about vulnerability, lack of ongoing safety, helplessness, and impaired sense of control. These beliefs—originating during trauma and based on limited cognitions, acute dependency, extreme fear, and realistic feelings of disempowerment—must be addressed precisely in a safe and structured environment. This type of work is not done in groups but in individual therapy; it is also begun only after a strong therapeutic relationship has been established, and the client has a well-defined sense of self, a repertoire of coping strategies, and an internal and external support system. The processing is not necessarily discrete, but may occur over a period of time. It is not necessary (or helpful) to review each and every abuse incident, but rather to select representative examples for exploration. The goals of trauma processing are (1) integration and reinterpretation of the event, and (2) resolution and closure regarding past events, so that the present and the future feel more in the individual's control.

There are various ways of assessing for traumatic impact, including the presence of chronic PTSD symptoms; active involvement with trauma material through behavioral reenactments; or symptomatology (e.g., ongoing anxiety or depression) that a client attributes to abuse experiences. In addition, individuals who are immersed in their past to the exclusion of their present or future, and who either avoid or are drawn to conversations that are abuse-focused, may be individuals with unresolved traumatic experiences.

When it becomes apparent to me—as it did in the following case example—that someone could benefit from an in-depth, structured processing of traumatic material, I explain the process, suggest its potential benefits, and offer an invitation to do the work.

CASE ILLUSTRATION

Susan was a 14-year-old Asian girl who had been sexually abused by her older brother, Steve, a number of times. The sudden and dramatic change in her behavior did not go undetected by her mother, who noted that Susan had stopped seeing her friends and had become reluctant to engage in physical activities. This was particularly odd, since Susan competed in gymnastics and had tournament aspirations. Although the mother was somewhat relieved because her daughter was now able to devote more of her time to her studies, she found her daughter's other behavior changes of concern.

Susan's reluctance to talk dissipated when her mother commented that she noticed that Susan was more relaxed when her brother, now in college, was away from home. Susan broke down and confided that Steve had molested her. Susan's mother did not bring her daughter for therapy, because she was concerned that her son would be punished. However, noticing her daughter's "sadness" and "worry," she suggested that Susan talk to the school counselor, who had been helpful to her in the past when she struggled to juggle her gymnastics and academic demands.

When Susan confided in the school counselor, she was stunned to discover that her counselor was required by law to report suspected child sexual abuse. Susan became frightened about her mother's reaction, and the school counselor interpreted Susan's concern for her mother as a sign that the mother was probably aware of what had happened and was unprotective. Susan was asked to stay in the office, the police were called, and she was taken to the police station. A discussion ensued about whether or not Susan could remain in her mother's custody, which threw Susan into tremendous despair. Since her father's tragic death in a car accident, Susan and her mother had been extremely close. The thought of living away from her mother was inconceivable.

Although Susan pleaded with the police to take her home, they instead sent an officer to the house to pick up Susan's mother and bring her to the police station – an act that frightened and humiliated the mother. When Susan and her mother were reunited, they talked in their first language (Chinese), which caused an officer to separate the mother and daughter unceremoniously. The officer later reported that he thought the two were "conspiring to make up a story to protect the perpetrator." Susan subsequently described her interrogation by the police and the disrespect shown toward her mother as one of her worst experiences – "a nightmare from start to finish." She added, "I honestly wish I had never said a word to the counselor, now that all this pain has been brought on my family."

Susan was bright and articulate. It was often difficult to separate the effects of the abuse from the impact of the interview process. She focused primarily on her mother's grief and felt responsible for bringing her shame and pain. The mother was inconsolable once she learned that her son would be arrested and could face a prison sentence. Her despair did not end when she learned that her son had been put on probation and ordered by the court to receive treatment. The mother blamed herself for not knowing a problem existed with her children, and her heart was heavy as she watched both her children struggle with their pain and confusion.

The mother was supportive of Steve's therapy and relieved that someone would help him with his problems. However, she was less convinced that Susan required therapy, and gave her mixed messages about the potential benefits of therapy. Nevertheless, she saw to it that Susan came to all of her appointments, often accompanying her back and forth on the bus so that her daughter would not feel alone.

After 6 months in therapy, Susan was unchanged. She continued to appear anxious, depressed, unresponsive, and uninterested in social or physical activities. She had insomnia, and on the rare occasions when she slept, she had nightmares that she never remembered but that produced cold sweats.

She talked with hesitancy about the sexual abuse, speaking in a flat monotone. She talked about herself as if she was talking about someone else; although she thought she should feel something about what had happened to her, she said she felt "numb, empty – sometimes I doubt whether it really occurred or it was a bad nightmare." Since Steve had readily admitted to sexually abusing Susan, I would often remind her that although it might feel like a bad dream, or she might wish it had never happened, her story was identical to what Steve had admitted. Discussions about Steve were very difficult for Susan.

She described total adoration of her brother, who had been like a father to her after her father's death. She talked dispassionately about how sweet and honorable he was, and how he would not hurt a fly. She talked about his many achievements, especially his early graduation from high school and the scholarship he had received to a top university. No emotion registered on her face as she spoke about Steve in glowing terms. She downplayed the sexual abuse, stating that he had been very gentle, had never hurt her, and had always seemed concerned for her comfort. "If I said 'no' he would have stopped – I know this – but I just couldn't say 'no' to him. I never have." Her belief that he would have stopped if she had asked him to, reinforced a myth that she was in control of whether or not the abuse occurred. Initially I responded, "Lots of girls who are sexually abused, particularly by family members they love, feel the way you do. . . if only they had said 'no,' if only they hadn't worn a certain blouse, if only they had done something to stop what was going on. Unfortunately, children don't have that much power when faced with someone they love and respect and want to please." This was a topic I would revisit later, but I approached it gingerly at first to avoid provoking resistance.

In the first 6 months in therapy, I had helped Susan identify and acknowledge her feelings. She seemed gradually more comfortable expressing herself to me, and she listened intently as I provided education on the topic of sexual abuse. She was very surprised to learn that sibling incest is not uncommon and that many teenagers experience sexual abuse. Up to this time, Susan had only heard about younger children being sexually abused, and only by their fathers.

She was very disappointed in the response of the legal system to her initial report, and failed to understand why the authorities had been so cruel and insensitive to her mother. When I suggested the possibility that the police might have thought that her mother had not been protective of her, she became enraged. She was angry at the disrespect with which they had treated her mother, whom she revered.

At the end of the first 6 months of treatment, I reviewed my initial goals with Susan, and she agreed that little change had occurred. "I don't know why I don't feel better," she stated. "I feel as if no time has gone by and it was just yesterday since he did those things to me." She had not seen Steve in the past 6 months, since his visiting home was prohibited by his probation. Steve had rented a room in his uncle's house and kept to himself, ashamed to face family or friends. The fact that she missed her brother, and was a witness to her mother's grief at not seeing her son, compounded Susan's predicament.

Here is a paraphrase of what I suggested to Susan at this juncture in the therapy:

> "Although you and I have talked about the sexual abuse, and you have been very clear about what Steve did to you–that is, what behavior was involved–I feel that there is a way in which you haven't yet felt whatever feelings you have about what happened. And because in some ways everything about the abuse has remained intact, just like the day it happened, you aren't able to put it in the past. It's almost as if these memories are frozen in time and place, and I believe it's helpful to thaw them out a little, so that they actually change in some way. Then they can be put in perspective."

Susan's first reactions were discomfort and curiosity. "How will you do that?" she asked quickly. "There's nothing magical about it," I said. "It just takes spending some time really talking about what happened."

"I feel I've been doing that for months."

"I know it must feel that way to you, but when you've talked about it, it's almost as if you were telling me about someone else."

"It does feel like it happened to another girl, not me."

"That's not unusual."

I then proceeded to explain to Susan the procedure we would follow, and invited her to participate when and if she was ready. This procedure is described in detail in the following section. However, with Susan's permission, I have transcribed a segment from an audiotape of this structured approach to processing traumatic material:

THERAPIST: So far, you've told me that you remember being in your bed, listening to noises outside your room, and then your brother turning the doorknob, coming over to your bed, getting in bed next to you, and putting his arms around you so that his hands fondle your breasts. Then you remember that he touches you for a while, pushes up against you, and then leaves.

SUSAN: Uh-huh, except that he also touches me down there.

THERAPIST: That's right. You told me he moves his hand down your pajamas, past your buttocks, and reaches over to your vagina.

SUSAN: Yes. (*Susan appears calm and detached.*)

THERAPIST: Now I would like to take this part that you've described so well, and see what else you remember about it.

SUSAN: Not much.

THERAPIST: Okay, let's just go through it slowly.

SUSAN: Okay.

THERAPIST: When you are in bed, you say you hear noises in the hallway. Some people may have some thoughts about what's going on, others may not. Any thoughts going on for you then?

SUSAN: Well, I know it's my mother, who has gotten up for her final trip to the bathroom. That means she's going to be asleep in the next 20 minutes.

THERAPIST: So what do you say to yourself?

SUSAN: "Uh-oh, she's going to sleep."

THERAPIST: Why "Uh-oh"?

SUSAN: Because then I know that's when Steve gets up.

THERAPIST: So your mother's final trip to the bathroom signals to everyone in the house that she will soon be sleeping, and Steve listens for that sign to come into your room.

SUSAN: Yes. I guess so.

THERAPIST: So you say, "Uh-oh, she's going to sleep." Anything else?

SUSAN: "Please, God, make Steve be asleep tonight."

THERAPIST: So you pray that he won't come to your room?

SUSAN: Yes, that he's already asleep.

THERAPIST: And when you say that little prayer, picture yourself in your mind's eye, and tell me what your body does.

SUSAN: My body?

THERAPIST: Yes. Just remember yourself in your bed and notice what your body does.

SUSAN: I bring my knees up to my chest.

THERAPIST: Anything else?

SUSAN: I don't think so.

THERAPIST: Where are your arms?

SUSAN: I fold them on my chest. (*Susan demonstrates, crossing her chest with her arms.*)

THERAPIST: Okay, and do you have any sensations in your body?

SUSAN: What do you mean?

THERAPIST: As you are lying there, knees to chest, arms folded over your chest, saying your little prayer that Steve remains asleep, do you have any physical sensations?

SUSAN: I feel kind of cold.

THERAPIST: All over?

SUSAN: Pretty much.

THERAPIST: And you've already said you're kind of listening for sounds in the hallway. Are there any sounds you notice now?

SUSAN: Just my heartbeat, loud in my ears.

THERAPIST: And is your heart beating fast?

SUSAN: Not really.

THERAPIST: And how is your breathing?

SUSAN: My breathing?

THERAPIST: Uh-huh . . . at that moment, with your knees to your chest, and your arms crossed over your chest, saying a prayer that Steve is asleep, and hearing your heart pounding in your ears . . .

SUSAN: I'm holding my breath.

THERAPIST: You're holding your breath . . .

SUSAN: So I can hear better.

THERAPIST: And how are you feeling right at that moment?

SUSAN: I guess I'm nervous.

THERAPIST: Try to picture yourself in that bed, at that moment, looking the way you do, with your body the way you've described, listening, praying . . .

SUSAN: I'm scared he's going to come in again.

THERAPIST: So would you say you might be feeling nervous or scared?

SUSAN: Yes.

THERAPIST: And how do you feel now talking about it?

SUSAN: Well, a little scared, like I remember that feeling right before.

THERAPIST: Good. You remember your feelings. You had them then, but you couldn't let them out. And even though they're not as strong now, and nothing bad is going to happen to you now, you can let your feelings out a little now. As a matter of fact, you can move your fingers and toes, you can move in your chair, and you can take a deep breath through your nose, and let out a big sigh through your mouth.

SUSAN: (*Takes a very deep breath, exhales, and shakes her hands.*) It feels good to move.

THERAPIST: Yes, although this may feel scary to remember, it is not something that's happening to you right now.

SUSAN: Okay.

THERAPIST: Let me know when you're ready to move on a little.

SUSAN: (*Taking some time, taking a sip of water, shaking her hands a little more*) I'm ready.

THERAPIST: Now the next thing I remember is that you said you see the doorknob move.

SUSAN: No, I don't see it, I hear it.

THERAPIST: I see. Which way are you facing, by the way?

SUSAN: Before, when I said I pulled my knees up, the other thing is that I turn around and face away from the door. I guess I don't want him to see me when he comes in.

THERAPIST: What happens if he sees you?

SUSAN: No, I mean sometimes, if he can't really see me, he thinks I'm sleeping and he leaves.

THERAPIST: Oh, I see. So you think you can pretend to be asleep better if he can't see your face.

SUSAN: Yeah, because I think my eyes move when I'm pretending.

THERAPIST: I see. So, in your own way, you're trying to signal him to stop.

SUSAN: I'm what?

THERAPIST: Well, you're trying to get him to believe that you're sleeping, so he won't get in bed with you. You're signaling him to stop.

SUSAN: I'm trying to trick him into leaving me alone.

THERAPIST: Yeah, pretty clever too.

SUSAN: Except it only works once in a while.

THERAPIST: You've never really said before, Susan, but how many times do you figure Steve molested you?

SUSAN: I know exactly. I counted.

THERAPIST: How many?

SUSAN: Thirteen different nights.

THERAPIST: And did he abuse you in the same way?

SUSAN: Mostly.

THERAPIST: Okay, we can talk about that as we go on, but let's get back to where we were. (*Pause*) Your back was turned away from the door, and in this specific time that you've chosen to work on today, does Steve leave or stay?

SUSAN: He stands there for a while, and then he picks up the sheet and climbs in on my back.

THERAPIST: What do you say to yourself at that point?

SUSAN: "God be with me."

THERAPIST: Another prayer.

SUSAN: Yes.

THERAPIST: Do you notice anything else, in your body, what you hear, what you feel?

SUSAN: Now my heartbeat goes really fast, and it's like a loud thumping in my ear. And I start counting.

THERAPIST: Counting?

SUSAN: I count my heartbeats.

THERAPIST: I see.

SUSAN: And my body goes limp, I guess because I'm pretending to be asleep. I just let go.

THERAPIST: And then?

SUSAN: He starts touching my chest . . . my nipples, he pinches them.

THERAPIST: And what happens?

SUSAN: I hate this part.

THERAPIST: What's that?

SUSAN: They get round and hard.

THERAPIST: Your nipples get round and hard?

SUSAN: Yeah.

THERAPIST: And how does it feel when he's pinching your nipples?

SUSAN: I don't like it. It hurts. And it makes me mad that my nipples get hard.

THERAPIST: Why does it make you mad?

SUSAN: Because I think he likes that.

THERAPIST: So you're mad that your body is reacting and that Steve likes what's happening.

SUSAN: Yeah . . .

THERAPIST: How do you feel talking about it now?

SUSAN: I feel mad.

THERAPIST: At Steve?

SUSAN: No, at my nipples.

THERAPIST: I see. Mad at your nipples for getting hard, but not mad at Steve, who is touching your nipples and getting them hard?

SUSAN: (*Laughs nervously*) I guess I'm a little mad at everybody.

THERAPIST: Everybody? Does that include Steve?

SUSAN: I guess, maybe.

THERAPIST: So your body is limp, and as usually happens, your nipples are reacting to getting pinched by becoming round and hard. And you're mostly mad at your body, your nipples, for reacting, but you're also maybe a little mad at Steve for touching your nipples.

SUSAN: Uh-huh.

THERAPIST: And what happens next?

SUSAN: The really bad part.

THERAPIST: What's that?

SUSAN: He goes inside my pants and he puts his fingers, you know . . .

THERAPIST: He puts one of his hands down your pajama pants?

SUSAN: Uh-huh.

THERAPIST: Do you always wear pajamas?

SUSAN: Before, I always wore a T-shirt.

THERAPIST: Before?

SUSAN: After the first time that it happened, I made my mom buy me some pajamas with a top and bottoms.

THERAPIST: So you stopped wearing a T-shirt and started wearing bottoms. How come?

SUSAN: I didn't want to make it easy for him.

THERAPIST: Oh, so here's another way you're trying to signal him to stop.

SUSAN: Well . . . Oh, I see. I wanted to make it hard on him to get down there.

THERAPIST: Right.

SUSAN: I never thought of that before.

THERAPIST: It's interesting the ways kids figure out to say no, even when they're not even aware they're saying no, or stop.

SUSAN: (A smile is quickly replaced by a frown.) A lot of good it did.

THERAPIST: Well, I tell you what. Kids try all kinds of things to make people stop hurting them, but people who molest children are usually pretty determined and they don't pay attention to kids' messages, because they're too busy worrying about what they want and how to get it.

SUSAN: I got wet down there, too.

THERAPIST: That happens sometimes. When the body is touched in certain places, certain reactions occur.

SUSAN: That was gross.

THERAPIST: How did you explain this wetness to yourself?

SUSAN: I didn't. I think it's gross.

THERAPIST: Well, it's what the body does when it's stimulated sexually, like when it's rubbed on the nipples.

SUSAN: I don't want to talk about this any more.

THERAPIST: That's fine, Susan. We can stop. You did a lot of work today, got a lot of new information. I know there are some things that are more difficult to talk about than others. Sex can feel funny to talk about. You can decide how much or little to say.

SUSAN: Okay. (Shaking her hands)

THERAPIST: Tell me how you're feeling now?

SUSAN: Okay, a little.

THERAPIST: Okay, just breathe deep, shake your hands, tell me how you're doing.

SUSAN: Well, I'm sort of glad we did this, because I remembered some stuff I didn't know.

THERAPIST: Like what?

SUSAN: Like buying my pajamas.

THERAPIST: Yeah, that was pretty resourceful of you.

SUSAN: It makes me think I wasn't so bad after all.

THERAPIST: How so?

SUSAN: Because, you know, I didn't, like, make it easy for him.

THERAPIST: You were trying to get him to stop.

SUSAN: Yeah.

THERAPIST: How does that make you feel?

SUSAN: I don't know.

THERAPIST: You're not sure how you feel, but you are sure it was important for you to know this.

SUSAN: Yeah.

THERAPIST: Good enough. You might have some more reactions to this later.

SUSAN: Yeah.

THERAPIST: Was anything surprising to you about what we did today?

SUSAN: Time went by fast!

THERAPIST: Yeah, that happens sometimes.

SUSAN: And . . . (Putting her hand over her mouth)

THERAPIST: Yes?

SUSAN: That I got mad at Steve.

THERAPIST: That's right. Mostly you were mad at your nipples, but yes, you let yourself get a little mad at Steve.

SUSAN: Yeah.

THERAPIST: And what surprised you about that?

SUSAN: I'm *never* mad at Steve.

THERAPIST: Really? You're never mad at your brother?

SUSAN: No, no.

THERAPIST: That's interesting. Most brothers and sisters I know get mad at each other a lot.

SUSAN: They're not Chinese, I bet.

THERAPIST: Well, let me think now. No, you know, I know two Chinese children who are 8 and 10, and they fight all the time.

SUSAN: They must be from this country.

THERAPIST: Yes.

SUSAN: Our way is to respect elders, honor family.

THERAPIST: I see. You've been taught to honor and respect Steve.

SUSAN: Always.

THERAPIST: You know, I have an older brother too, and we Latins are taught the same thing—honor and respect elders. I remember once I caught him cheating at cards. Wow! I didn't know what to think, because here was my older brother who could do no wrong, and he had done something that was not worthy of honor or respect.

SUSAN: Steve is always honorable.

THERAPIST: Even honorable people make mistakes sometimes.

SUSAN: I guess.

THERAPIST: Have you talked to Steve after the abuse happened?

SUSAN: I haven't seen him since then. First he left the house because he was ashamed, and later the probation person said he had to stay away.

THERAPIST: And you miss him?

SUSAN: Very much.

THERAPIST: And your mother?

SUSAN: She cries every day from missing him.

THERAPIST: When will he return?

SUSAN: We don't know.

THERAPIST: Well, at some later time, after we get through this work we're doing now, we'll talk about my meeting with Steve or talking to his therapist, and maybe you and he coming together to talk about what happened.

SUSAN: You mean Steve and I would talk about it?

THERAPIST: Yes.

SUSAN: I can't imagine that.

THERAPIST: I understand. Nothing will happen before you are ready and without your permission.

SUSAN: Okay.

This session was followed by two additional sessions in which we took selected memories and processed them in similar fashion. Susan responded very well to these sessions, and when she reported having nightmares about the abuse, I reframed this as a good sign: "When you are sleeping, all your defenses are down, and things come up that need your attention. Dreams point us to things we need to look at."

Susan felt fortified through this process and looked forward to seeing her brother again. I have never forgotten a statement she made just before we went into the first sibling session. Susan looked at me pointedly and said, "The last time Steve saw me I was a little girl. Now he's going to hear from the woman."

Steve's therapy had been very successful, and he was able to apologize earnestly for the mistakes he had made – exploiting her innocence, violating her trust, and intruding into her sexual development. When he cried, Susan comforted him and forgave him profusely, but added, "You were wrong to do this, and I forgive you."

His open expression of shame did not deter her from telling him what she had learned about the sexual abuse, how she had felt, how it had affected her and her mother, and how she wanted him to continue in therapy so he would never hurt anyone again.

STEPS IN STRUCTURED PROCESSING OF TRAUMA

Assessing Readiness

In my experience, the processing of trauma-related material is best done in individual therapy, utilizing a structured, time-limited approach. I have not found it useful to attempt this type of sensitive work in groups, although I hear from trusted colleagues that they have done this type of work with adolescents who feel safer in a group and are better able to utilize the support of their peers.

Several factors must precede this type of structured work. First, there should be a strong therapeutic relationship, in which both parties feel there is emotional connectedness, trust, respect, and communication. Within the context of a strong therapeutic relationship, the therapist's opinions are valued, suggestions are followed, and there is a general willingness to reveal inner thoughts and feelings. There is no exact time period for forming such a relationship; in my experience, depending on the individual's motivation for treatment, openness, and ability to trust the therapy process, a strong enough relationship can be developed within 3 months of starting weekly therapy sessions. For individuals with histories of severe abuse and neglect, this time frame must be extended, since their abilities to be open, trustful, motivated, and comfortable in the context of a personal relationship have probably been compromised by their experiences of abuse and neglect. I have worked with individuals who still feel like "new" clients even after 2 or 3 years in therapy.

Equally important to the decision of whether to proceed with trauma processing is the therapist's evaluation of the client's ego strength, coping strategies, and ability to identify and use an external support system. Within this area, the therapist must feel confident that the individual has a broad repertoire of coping strategies, can adequately gauge his or her pain thresholds, can decrease his or her feelings of anxiety and pain, can create a sense of internal and external comfort and safety, has personal power (i.e., can agree or disagree to follow suggestions), and has the ability to pace difficult material.

Preparing/Informing the Clients: Making the Invitation

Once the therapist believes that a client can benefit from and can tolerate a structured and focused approach to working on past abuse, he or she informs the client about what the process involves. Earlier in this chapter, I have paraphrased what I usually say to clients when I believe they are good candidates for engaging in this procedure. It is important to demystify this therapy process by emphasizing its potential value and its short-term, structured nature.

Often clients jump to conclusions about how painful this process may be, or how overwhelmed they may feel. They also may suspect that the therapist will be "doing" something to them that will jeopardize their personal control. The therapist must make clear that the client is always in control of how much or how little is said, how much is remembered or revealed, or when to stop or continue the flow of work. In order to promote my clients' feeling of personal power or control in therapy, I always *invite* the clients to do this work, asking them to consider what I've said to them about how this type of structured focus may be valuable to them.

Obtaining a Contract for the Work

The next step is to obtain a contract that specifies what will be done, for how long, and toward what end. Below is one version of such a contract, signed by Susan and myself:

> I, _____, accept the invitation to spend no more than five sessions thinking about, remembering, and talking about past events of childhood abuse. I understand that these sessions will run longer

than the usual 50 minutes (90 minutes) and that I may be asked to come in more than once a week while the work is underway. I also understand that I can stop this process at any time if it becomes too stressful, or it is not useful, and also that I can extend it for a couple more sessions if it seems helpful to me. The purpose of doing this work is to focus on these events so they may be better understood, and so that any feelings left unfelt or any words left unspoken may find expression. The ultimate goals of this work are to put the abuse finally behind me, to put it in proper perspective, and to understand it fully.

Obviously, contracts can be tailored to an individual's specific needs. Clients may sometimes postpone the work, but it is rare when someone chooses to discontinue the work permanently.

Selecting Traumatic Incidents for Recall

Although there is a great deal of controversy not only about the way individuals access memories of abuse, but the accuracy of those memories, my experience has shown me that traumatized individuals often remember many details of their abuse years after they occurred. As a matter of fact, for many traumatized individuals memories seem almost intact, as if they happened yesterday.

Obviously, for others this is not the case. A small percentage of adult survivors whom I have treated cannot access specific memories of abuse, and remain frustrated and concerned that they cannot remember details to support their intuitive feelings that something frightening and unsettling happened to them when they were children. Still others have an adult experience (e.g., marriage, birth of a child, death of a parent, or some other apparently unrelated event) that triggers a memory, or creates a bridge between a current event or stimulus and the past.

One adult survivor in her 50s sought therapy when she walked into her apartment and discovered that burglars had broken in, slitting her mattress in half, emptying all her drawers, and painting graffiti on the wall. When she witnessed this horrible scene, she felt violated – a feeling that apparently caused her to have an abrupt, intrusive memory of having been raped when she was 4 years old. Disturbed by this memory, which seemed dislodged by witnessing the burglary scene and having the feeling of violation, she called a sister to ask whether she remembered any such childhood event. Her sister, 8 years older, verified that in fact my client had been raped at age 4 and that the family had felt the wisest and most helpful thing to do was never to speak of the rape again. It might have remained a dormant memory had it not been jarred by the events of the burglary.

In therapy, this woman was able to use her intrusive memory as a stepping stone to other fragments of memory, such as the fact that her mouth had been covered, and that she had smelled the smell of garbage during the rape. Her sister confirmed that the family had been on an outing at a carnival, which had been set up on an empty lot; that my client had wandered away; and that a man had dragged her into an alley, where there were many full garbage cans nearby. A passer-by screamed, which caused the rapist to flee and my client to be rescued from what could possibly have been a rape/murder.

When I work with adolescents, there is the added advantage that the abuse memories are more "fresh" than the memories of adult survivors. Most adolescents remember instances of physical and sexual abuse, or acute or chronic episodes of psychological maltreatment or neglect, all too well. Like Susan, however, many adolescents believe wrongly that if they don't think or talk about their past abuse, then they will automatically feel better, and the abuse won't have negative repercussions. Unfortunately, this is rarely the case, especially when the abuse has had a traumatic impact on the individual.

Once a client agrees to engage in trauma processing, the client is then asked to choose a specific memory – vague or clear, as the case may be – for exploration. I tell clients, "You may choose a memory of the first time it happened, or the last time, or any time in between that held some significance for you." Obviously, if clients do not reveal a history of childhood abuse, such a question is inappropriate and intrusive. But in many adolescent abuse cases, as I have mentioned earlier, youngsters either describe their abuse in great detail or insist that the abuse that did occur had very little importance to them. In other words, they are more likely to deny the impact of the abuse than they are to deny the facts.

If a client has difficulty choosing, I encourage him or her to rate memories of specific incidents of abuse on a scale of 0–10. Zero means "no difficulty," while 10 is "very difficult" to remember or talk about. I then ask them to choose a memory in the range of 1–3. Starting with nonthreatening material is almost always best and allows the client to build up tolerance for the work.

Assisting with Assimilation of Experiences

As described in the case of Susan, youngsters may remember their abuse experiences in a fragmented way. The best metaphor I can give for this is of a mirror that has received a single jolt and is shattered into small pieces (see Figure 1). The shattered mirror represents a traumatic event for a youngster who has limited cognitive, physical, and emotional resources. The event is overwhelming and therefore cannot be easily reassembled and assimilated.

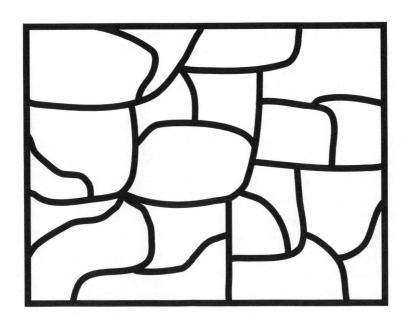

FIGURE 1

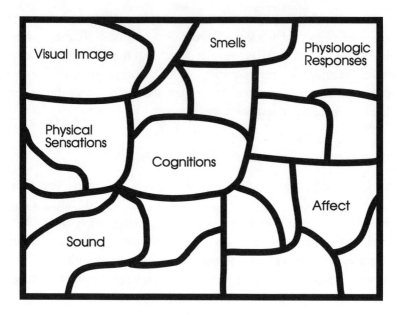

FIGURE 2

The next illustration (Figure 2) shows that each of these frag-ments contains pockets of information regarding an event – pockets of information kept separate by walls or barriers. Bloch (1991) describes dissociation as a process of separating or compartmentalizing discrete pieces of information such as thoughts and perceptions. Dis-sociation is strongly linked to trauma, and indeed is viewed as a com-mon defense against trauma. It is likely, then, that dissociative barriers confine aspects of an event to specific fragments, thus keeping a trau-matic memory chaotic, segmented, and without resolution.

And yet many of these pockets of information can become avail-able if individuals focus on them. Focusing on these fragmented or segregated aspects of an event allows for integration, or breaking down of dissociative barriers. As information becomes integrated, the individual can slowly tolerate more and more information, and can also now process it with a fuller cognitive range. The individu-al can reassess earlier views or perceptions; this often leads to feel-ings of mastery. Susan, for example, was relieved and pleased to understand that there were many ways in which she had tried to say "no" through her behavior, even though she was not able to verbalize "no" to her brother.

I must emphasize that the goal of reviewing or processing this material is not to elicit abreaction (i.e., the release of repressed emotions). Again, the goal of reviewing or processing this material in this purposeful way is to achieve integration, which tends to transform the memory and result in feelings of power and mastery.

Most individuals recall several content areas or aspects of the event; however, it is common for traumatized individuals to continue to keep some material out of conscious awareness, and it is not necessary to encourage or insist on obtaining full recall. In doing this work, I am informed by research on memory: Perry (1987) states that children often remember sensorimotor information (e.g., how things smell and taste), and that children under the age of 7 often take "snapshots" of events that have particular meaning to them. This information is helpful, because in many instances the traumatic experiences occurred when our adolescent or adult clients were children, not the individuals we see before us in treatment now. Because of this, I make sure to inquire about sounds, smells, and sensations, and I always ask what an individual sees or focuses on.

Perry (1987) also states that to assist in the process of having children recall and recount abuse experiences, reconstructive tasks are useful. On occasion, as I have documented elsewhere (Gil, 1988), I offer props to help individuals reconstruct what happened to them. Adolescents have responded particularly well when I've offered them miniature people, dollhouses, or puppets as props that assist their communication. In an interesting way, since so many adolescents are familiar with the sort of dissociative experiences that they describe as "floating overhead," they find it easy to engage with concrete objects, observing them from a third-party stance. One 15-year-old girl, who had been given an anatomically complete doll as a prop, placed the doll on a bed in front of her and said, "Oh, yeah. I remember I used to curl up like this, and over here [she used an available prop] was a lamp I used to stare at while he was doing shit to me." Amazingly, this youngster then felt propelled to draw a large image

of a lamp, paying special attention to the design on the lampshade –
rows of horses racing. "I would imagine I was on the horse that
was winning, and I would hold on tight and ride and ride, faster
than the wind, with my hair blowing in the wind, and we would
always win." Then the girl noted, with surprise, "I guess this is when
I first developed my love for horses." She had a huge collection of
miniature horses.

Encouraging Discharge of Affect

Although abreaction is not the goal of this work, it is frequently
one of the experiences that traumatized individuals find helpful. If
we use the metaphor provided above of the fragments kept separate
by dissociative barriers, we can understand why we often encoun-
ter adolescents who talk about their abuse experiences as if they happened to someone else and not to them. Obviously, the information
about the behavior that occurred, and the feelings associated with
the events, are kept separate from each other.

And yet releasing feelings that were perhaps not consciously felt,
or were walled off during traumatic events, may lead the person
to experience relief. The release of feelings that could not be safely
released earlier may be empowering and rewarding. Therefore, even
though abreaction is not the focus, and affect is often difficult for
adolescents to acknowledge or express, it is valuable to keep inviting an exploration of affect. Questions such as "How did you feel
about that?" or "What do you think you might have been feeling
at that point?" may encourage the individual to sort out and express
a range of emotions.

It is important never to suggest a discrete affect in a leading way.
A question such as "You probably felt really scared, didn't you?"
not only suggests the therapist's interpretation of how the client felt;
it also encourages compliance with that interpretation. A better way
to pose the question may be to help the client *reflect* on how he or
she might have felt: "So far you've told me your heart was beating
fast, your knees were curled up, and you were biting the inside of
your lip and swallowing your blood. As you see yourself in your

mind's eye, in that position, knowing what was about to happen, how do you imagine you might have felt?" If the youngster is still unable to identify feelings, the therapist should give him or her more distance: "As you think of any child, in the dead of night, pretending to be asleep, hoping and praying he won't get abused that night, and he pretends to be asleep, and his body goes numb, how do you think a child like that might feel?" If the client is still unable to provide verbal responses, he or she can be asked to point to a poster with expressions on it, or to draw a picture of the feeling, or simply to engage in further exploration on this subject. Finally, a therapist who chooses to suggest feelings to a client should be sure to suggest a range of feelings, never just one: "Some children who have had similar experiences have told me they have felt scared, nervous, sad, or angry, and some of them feel bad because they think they're doing something wrong. Do any of those feelings ring a bell for you?"

The releasing of feelings can be helpful to many people. However, it is equally useful to help young clients with affect tolerance. They need to have the ability to "sit with" their feelings so they can learn that their feelings will not overwhelm or consume them, and they also need to know how to comfort themselves so that they can build a repertoire of strategies, or internal resources, that they will use throughout their lives (see Chapter Four).

Sequencing the Information Provided by the Client

As youngsters provide information, it is useful to collect and organize it so that it becomes sequential. This type of order encourages feelings of mastery. The memory is no longer fragmented and nonsensical, without a beginning, middle, or end. It takes shape, becoming better organized and less chaotic; this permits it to be assimilated more easily.

Distinguishing the Past from the Present and Future

I believe one of the most useful interventions during this work is to distinguish among what happened in the past, what happens in the present, and what can happen in the future. In particular, this is an opportunity to honor the defenses of the past while acknowledging the current or future defenses as well. Susan, for example, came to an important conclusion regarding behavior that had caused her to reproach herself:

> "When I was younger, my brother was like a god to me. I would never have thought of saying no to him about anything. I looked up to him so much that I could never question anything he did. I've grown up now. I see him through more grownup eyes, and I can see he is just a human, and he makes mistakes like we all do . . . well, maybe bigger than most."

Helping Susan realize that her inability to say "no" to her brother was related to the nature of their relationship, and to her dependent status, served as a major source of comfort for her. This cognitive reassessment of her behavior allowed her to be more self-accepting, and probably motivated her to become assertive with others, instead of having "blind faith" in them.

Often I have worked with adolescents who think of their ability to dissociate or "space out" as something weird or unusual. I try to honor this defense by normalizing it and making it user-friendly. I'll often tell kids, "What a neat trick you pulled, that you were able to get yourself out of that difficult situation, and not feel uncomfortable feelings." At the same time, I think it's important for them to have additional resources. "Nowadays," I'll continue, "you know you can space out when you want to, but you also know that you can handle your difficult feelings in a number of new ways."

Yvonne Dolan (1991) has talked about concrete symbols that represent the past or present for individuals who are working on difficult past issues. This idea has been particularly helpful for adolescents, who respond very well to objects they can take home – objects that represent transitions of some kind. For example, I was working with an adolescent boy of 14 on the fact that he had been sexually abused by a neighbor when he was 9 years old. He was particularly resistant to talking about what had happened to him, and yet remained encopretic, self-injurious, and anxious. I gave him a metaphor he understood:

> "When there's something in the shadows and you don't know what it is, and it's making noises, and you're afraid of it, what do you do? Do you keep the lights off, let the noises get louder, without taking any more steps to see what it is? Or do you turn the lights on, look at what's in the corner, and then decide what to do? Would it be different if it was a cricket or a mouse? Would it be different if it was a toy that was left on with a dwindling battery? What if it was a bat, or a small kitten? Would it be more helpful if you had an adult who would go with you and turn on the light for you? And how would you respond if you found some of the different things I've mentioned so far?"

Finally the boy understood that his sexual abuse was in the shadows, and it made noises that scared him in the night, but he was afraid to go turn on the light. But as long as the light was turned off, he couldn't see. I told him that I would go with him and stay by his side when he turned on the light, and then he could see what was there and deal with it. I gave this boy a very small flashlight, which represented light that he could shine on difficult past events. He carried the flashlight with him for a couple of months before he stated, "I think I'm okay to look at the shadows now." Then we did the work described in this chapter; it was difficult for him, but restored his sense of safety and security in the long run.

Challenging Idiosyncratic Meaning

Many individuals with abuse in their past find specific elements of their abuse experiences particularly momentous for a variety of reasons. Often a critical aspect of how an abusive experience is addressed depends on the idiosyncratic meaning a client attributes to the event. For example, one adolescent told me, "This always happens to me. People can sense that I won't put up a fight – they see me as an easy target." Further exploration revealed that this youngster's belief system about her own lack of personal power had originated when she was sexually abused between the ages of 4 and 6. When her original abuse by her father was discovered, she was placed in foster care until her mother was able to provide for her. During her foster placement, she was abused by an older foster child.

During the original abuse, this youngster's father told my client that he was putting his fingers inside her vagina because she was a good little girl, and good little girls always get loved in special ways. The older child who abused her in foster care reinforced this message by telling her she was very good and had special powers to make him feel good. Both the child's father and the older foster child rewarded her by paying attention to her and giving her gifts for being good.

My client's older sister had also been sexually abused. However, their father had a preference for younger children, so that when his older daughter turned 10 he no longer pursued her sexually, turning instead to my client, then 4 years old. The 10-year-old daughter became the family scapegoat and was frequently banished to her room or physically punished. My client was repeatedly told that her sister was bad, and that bad children should not be seen or heard. My client feared being rejected by her father, particularly since her mother was an alcoholic who spent much of her time sleeping or crying. Since my client longed for attention and affection, she was afraid to be anything but compliant when her father sexually abused her. She therefore learned through repeated confirmations that she was a sexual object, valued only for her physical compliance. She was stripped of personal power and a sense of entitlement, and her self-esteem remained understandably paltry.

Another adolescent client agonized over her final and most profound secret. She was racked with ambivalence about whether or not to tell me. Some days she would come in, sit down, and announce that today she was going to tell me this final secret; however, it took many false starts before she was able to confide in me. As a matter of fact, she put her secret on a tape recorder, and after bringing it to therapy for at least eight sessions, she left the tape recorder behind. Calling me that evening to make sure I wouldn't listen to it, she called back later to say that she wanted me to listen to it before our next session. Of course, she missed our next session. I called during the hour to find her at home, anxious about whether or not I had listened to the tape. I told her that I had listened to it, and that I wanted to talk to her about it so I could better understand her feelings; I told her I would wait for her to come in (she lived about 5 minutes from my office and rode her bike quickly to our sessions). Apparently, my asking her to come over immediately was very important to her, since her biggest fear about my finding out about the secret was that I would no longer want to see her in treatment (and that, in fact, I would consider her a phony).

To make a very long story short, this youngster had been sexually abused by a camp counselor during summer camp. Although we had worked on this experience and it was my impression that she was now less burdened by the occurrence, she had never mentioned that the camp counselor had only one leg. When we finally talked it over, it became clear that she had given this fact undue importance: She believed that since he had only one leg, this meant that she could have gotten away from him if she had really made an effort. We reviewed the circumstances (she had been tied down, stripped, and orally violated), and she was able to acknowledge that she had made many efforts to get away, but the young man had tremendous upper body strength and had overpowered her. Once we talked it over, she adjusted her perception of the event and was able to release herself from feelings of guilt and shame brought on by her faulty idiosyncratic perception.

I don't usually confront idiosyncratic beliefs directly. If someone tells me that something happened because he or she was bad, I will always ask, "What did you do or say that made you bad?" This allows the client to communicate hidden perceptions of the event. Once the client tells me something—for example, "I was bad because I didn't tell someone right away"—then I usually explore this belief gently, by asking questions such as these: "What might have gotten in the way of your telling someone?" "Who would have been most upset by what you had to say?" "What do you think your mother [father, teacher, etc.] might have done or said if you told her [him]?" "What was the most important thing you wanted to tell someone?" These questions will usually elicit the youngster's expectations of others, and perhaps less defined fears or concerns as well. I may summarize: "So there were lots of very strong reasons that got in your way at that point in your life, and perhaps at this point, equipped with what you know now, you might view and overcome those obstacles in different ways."

Emphasizing Transformations

Once youngsters do this work, they, in essence, "take the bull by the horns." In other words, whatever resistance they may feel about discussing past traumatic events will almost immediately decrease. There is simply no way to focus on these events, process them in this manner, and verbalize the unspoken without transforming clients' memories of them. Events that have been foreboding, overwhelming, or controlling become less potent, charged, vibrant, or intrusive in the clients' minds.

I usually make explicit what I notice. For example, Susan literally shook in her seat when we first discussed her brother, so riddled with guilt and fear was she by the idea of betraying family confidences. As the memories were transformed through this structured, in-depth exploration, they seemed less powerful to her. It was wonderful to watch her take back her personal power and control. I would often remark that there was a clear difference in her physical posture, tone of voice, and general appearance between her earlier and later discussions of the sexual abuse.

Encouraging Understanding of Skills
Used during the Work

Clients and therapists are often too quick to mystify the process of therapy. I like clients to understand fully what helps them, either in what I do or in what they do. Therefore, I ask clients to think about what it is I say or do that is helpful, or what it is about the process of therapy that they find valuable. When specific variables are identified, clients are encouraged to utilize these skills outside the therapy hour.

Preparing the Client to Leave the Therapy Sessions

Some clients feel more or less disoriented after focusing intently on specific events that elicit difficult memories, sensations, or thoughts. It is therefore important to have longer sessions (as noted earlier, I suggest 90 minutes), so that the last half hour can be used for re-orienting a client to the room, and later to the larger environment. During this time it is useful to talk about what clients will do for the rest of the day, how they will take care of themselves, whom they will call if they need to talk, what they will do if they have more thoughts about the session (I recommend they write things down for the following session), and what they can expect in the next session.

Giving Cognitive Tasks

If individuals state their fears about crying too much, having night-mares, feeling depressed, or the like, it may be useful to discuss what to do when and if these circumstances arise. I often help clients come up with ideas about cognitive tasks to undertake when specific feared events come up. For example, if clients are afraid of having night-mares, we can discuss something for them to do when they wake up from a nightmare, such as writing down as much as they remem-ber about images, colors, content, and so forth. Some clients make audiotapes that they listen to when they are feeling out of sorts or frightened; the tapes reassure them and stabilize them in a very im-portant way. Sometimes clients tape their therapy sessions and find that it is comforting to listen to them during the week.

Discussing Self-Care

Lastly, depending on a client's specific style of working, it is useful to discuss what the client already knows about initiating reparative experiences. Although many people know the things that help them feel better, it is during difficult times that these items seem more elusive. Therefore, making a list of "what to do to help myself," or "what to do to take care of myself," may be a useful resource in the future, and can definitely be beneficial during this work. These lists include activities, as well as contact with people who provide unconditional love and acceptance.

Trauma resolution work is necessary when individuals have unresolved traumatic experiences. Some individuals seem able to resolve these life experiences on their own, or with the help of extended family or friends. In particular, when there is an appropriate, nurturing, and protective nonabusive parent, this serves as a strong factor in mitigating long-term negative consequences of abuse. Conversely, when youngsters not only endure abuse by one parent, but do not have another parent to demonstrate love and safety, the impact of the abuse may be more long-lasting. In addition, when abuse is severe, chronic, bizarre, and perpetrated by a loved family member, the potential for traumatic impact increases.

ADVANTAGES OF STRUCTURED PROCESSING

Processing traumatic material in this structured, time-limited, focused way has many potential rewards, including the following:

- It makes affect available for treatment.
- It provides the client with a clearer understanding of the idiosyncratic meaning of abuse, and allows for cognitive reassessments of previous belief systems.
- It makes previously intolerable thoughts, memories, and sensations more tolerable, therefore diffusing the power of unresolved traumatic memories.
- It organizes material and allows for a less chaotic or fragmented view of prior life experiences.
- It results in less need for dissociative responses.
- It allows the client to go from passivity of intrusive memories, or unconscious behavioral reenactments, to controlled recall.
- It allows for conscious processing – that is, for insight and understanding.
- It restores feelings of mastery and control.
- It instills hope in the future and shifts the client to a future orientation.

- It frees up energy that has heretofore been tied up with unresolved trauma, and allows that energy to be used in the productive pursuit of life interests, including relationships with others.

COUNTERINDICATIONS AND SAFEGUARDS

Any time therapy involves issues that are highly likely to be painful and troubling for individuals, it must proceed carefully.

I define this process as time-limited and structured, in order to relieve some anxiety about how long it may take or what it may entail. As I have mentioned earlier, I demystify what the process involves, and I explain the steps involved in the work. I do not convey an expectation that the work will be debilitating or overwhelming; in fact, I talk about pacing and the goal of mastery and control. I expect that this process will produce the desired results – specifically, that individuals will disengage from the past and begin to focus on the present and the future with a renewed sense of control and competence.

It is important, however, to avoid "flooding," in which individuals are overwhelmed by their affect. As a matter of fact, part of what is helpful about structuring this process is the individual's gradual exposure to anxiety-producing material, which is thus better tolerated and can produce a sense of accomplishment and empowerment.

If adolescents become despondent, disoriented, acutely depressed, or generally unable to function, obviously the work must cease immediately, and crisis intervention strategies designed to stabilize the young clients must be provided. Suicidal or homicidal thoughts or feelings must be carefully assessed as well. On occasion, I have had adult survivors feel rageful feelings and develop homicidal ideation. In these cases, creating safety for the clients (and their intended victims) must take precedence over the structured work.

Substance use and abuse must be evaluated carefully as well. My experience suggests that it is important not to undertake trauma-processing work until a substance-abusing client has been in recovery for at least 1 year. Often, addressing past issues provokes instability in the recovery process. Likewise, if adolescents use drugs as a result of (or prior to coming to) sessions that are structured to work on unresolved trauma, they are signaling their inability or unwillingness to participate at this time. I respect the youngsters' action language and hold off until another, more appropriate time.

Although I believe in the power of this process to help individuals with unresolved trauma that is interfering with current functioning, not everyone benefits from it. I make certain that each client understands the purpose, has given informed consent, and knows that he or she can ask for the process to cease at any time. This is not a process I impose on people; rather, it is a process that they cooperate with, in the hope that it will relieve them of painful (dormant) material that is creating difficulties in their current functioning. The overriding goal is to help them achieve a sense of control over traumatic events, acknowledge the past, and move on to the sculpting of a productive life.

THE THERAPIST'S STANCE

Finally, the therapist's stance throughout the process of structured trauma-processing is worth noting. The therapist must be physically fortified and emotionally present in order to assist the client. This means that when clinicians undertake this work they should be well-rested, well-nourished, and enjoying low stress and emotional well-being. Your role as witness cannot be overemphasized. Your unconditional acceptance of the client's dignity must remain intact.

Herman (1992) says it best: "The therapist normalizes the patient's responses, facilitates naming and the use of language, and shares the emotional burden of the trauma. She also contributes to constructing a new interpretation of the traumatic experience that affirms the dignity and value of the survivor. . . . As the therapist listens, she must constantly remind herself to make no assumptions about either the facts or the meaning of the trauma to the patient" (p. 179). Our clients trust us with delicate and painful information and our participation is a privilege as well as an opportunity to help.

CHAPTER SIX

General Principles in Working with Abused Adolescents

The following general principles are useful in therapeutic approaches with generic clients, but optimize the creation of therapeutic trust with abused adolescent clients.

TAKING A NONJUDGMENTAL ATTITUDE/POSTURE

Adolescents seem to be acutely sensitive to adults' judgments about their behavior. Perhaps because this is a period in which differentiation is expectable and control issues are ripe for negotiation, youngsters seem to have special antennae to detect any semblance of negativity from adults.

When an adolescent is referred to me because of a problem behavior, I do two things immediately: I support the intent of the behavior and reframe it as something potentially useful to the young client (see below), and I try to ascertain whether there are ways in which the behavior is a problem to the client. I always refrain from directing youngsters to stop doing something even if their ceasing a particular behavior is my ultimate goal. From experience, I know that my directives to do or not to do certain things may result in exactly the opposite of what I desire. As a matter of fact, because of the predictable resistance from many adolescents who come to treatment, paradoxical interventions are often effective ones.

Amos was a 14-year-old African-American youngster who had been sexually abused by his maternal grandmother. He was very aggressive toward peers and authority figures, and he was referred to therapy because his conduct in the classroom was becoming increasingly disruptive. Amos had been placed in his current foster care when he was 10 years old and had an ambivalent relationship with his foster parents, seemingly resenting them for being part of the system that had originally removed him from his mother and placed him in his grandmother's care. Interestingly, this young man did not consider the sexual abuse by his grandmother "a big deal," stating that he had been sexually active a long time before the grandmother "sucked me off." It was difficult to know for sure whether Amos was indeed unaffected by his grandmother's sexual conduct with him, or whether he was as sexually knowledgeable and experienced as he reported.

His social worker reviewed his records and informed me that Amos's mother was a very young prostitute who had given birth to Amos when she was 13. Amos's early history included numerous foster placements and failed rehabilitation attempts for the mother. The mother used her earnings to buy liquor, apparently minimizing her substance dependence because it was confined to alcohol. The mother's history also revealed her own sexual abuse at age 10, and a history of growing up in foster homes and group homes. She finally ran away and could not be located when she was 12. She resurfaced when Amos was born, and the protective services and health departments were called upon to assist her. Unfortunately, the mother was unable to secure a place to live, the paternal grandmother was unavailable to care for Amos because of physical illness, and he was placed in the first of a long series of foster placements. Although relative placements were sought at the outset, Amos's maternal grandmother was not willing to be his caretaker until he was older; this placement was short-lived due to Amos's allegation of sexual abuse.

Given the amount of instability in Amos's young life, the fact that he had only recently gotten in trouble at school was remarkable. My guess was that the fact that he had had a stable foster placement for the last 4 years had mitigated some of the possible long-term effects of his early instability and abuse. Although the records did not reveal specific incidents of abuse during periods with his mother, several notes reflected the mother's ongoing prostitution and alcoholism, with the possibility that Amos witnessed his mother's activities. Certainly his own references to being sexually knowledgeable at an early age may have had something to do with his environment.

Amos was a reluctant client. He stated early in therapy that he didn't know why he had to come see me and he wasn't doing anything that everybody else in his school didn't do. Below is an excerpt from our first meeting, which illustrates the importance of being nonjudgmental and nonpunitive.

THERAPIST: I hear you, Amos. You think it's a drag to have to come here.

AMOS: Yeah, I do.

THERAPIST: And there's probably lots of other things you could be doing right now.

AMOS: Damn straight.

THERAPIST: And you're not even sure why you're here.

AMOS: That's right.

THERAPIST: You haven't got a clue . . .

AMOS: I didn't say that.

THERAPIST: Well, fill me in, then. What happened that you got sent to see me?

AMOS: The teacher has it out for me. She thinks everything I do is wrong. She's always picking on my butt.

THERAPIST: So your teacher notices every little thing you do.

AMOS: Yeah.

THERAPIST: Can you give me an example of that?

AMOS: Like last Friday. Me and my friends were hanging out together, like talking, that's all, and then she yells, "Yo, Amos, this is the last time I tell you to quit talking and distracting everybody else." Like it was only me, like I was talking to myself.

THERAPIST: So there you were, talking to your buddies, and you get singled out.

AMOS: That's right.

THERAPIST: And then what happened?

AMOS: I told her to get off my back, and she sent me to the principal's office, like I care.

THERAPIST: So first she singled you out, told you to stop talking, and then you told her to get off your back. Is that right?

AMOS: Well, she was up on my case for a while.

THERAPIST: What do you mean?

AMOS: She says, "Amos, I'm up to here with this and that," and then she comes over and gets right in my face.

THERAPIST: Oh, so you had a few more words after she singled you out?

AMOS: I'm not gonna sit there and take her bull. Just because she's a teacher don't mean she can just ride all over my back.

THERAPIST: How do you feel right now, Amos?

AMOS: It pisses me off.

THERAPIST: What pisses you off?

AMOS: The way she's on my case all the time. Like I'm the only one who does anything while she's up there boring us out.

THERAPIST: And what do you do with your pissed-off feelings when you get them?

AMOS: I don't know. She just ticks me off.

THERAPIST: You feel like she picks on you, makes it seem that you're the only one doing something wrong.

AMOS: Yeah, and I'm not. There's lots of kids bullshitting all the time, but she's got Amos to shit on, so that's what she does.

THERAPIST: Does she ever single you out for anything you do right?

AMOS: Hell, no.

THERAPIST: Hm. I wonder why not?

AMOS: I told you. She's got it out for me. Maybe she doesn't like black kids.

THERAPIST: You think she picks on you because you're black.

AMOS: She doesn't pick on any white kids in the class.

THERAPIST: And you're the only black kid she picks on?

AMOS: Yeah, well, mostly . . . I mean, sometimes my buddies get in trouble too.

THERAPIST: So she picks on other black kids.

AMOS: Yeah, but no whities though.

THERAPIST: Never?

AMOS: Never that I can tell.

THERAPIST: Is she black?

AMOS: No, she's white too.

THERAPIST: Too?

AMOS: Like you.

THERAPIST: Were you surprised that I was white?

AMOS: Nah. I figured I'd have to see a white counselor.

THERAPIST: Why did you figure that?

AMOS: 'Cuz I saw one before, when I was little. She was white too.

THERAPIST: And how did you like your counselor when you were little?

AMOS: She was cool.

THERAPIST: Good. I'm glad you had someone cool to help you.

AMOS: She was all right.

THERAPIST: And back to the classroom, and your teacher. Have you ever been able to tell her, or your principal, that you feel you're getting picked on?

AMOS: Nobody listens to me.

THERAPIST: I'm listening. And from what you're describing, it must be really hard to feel like someone's picking at you all the time, and I can imagine getting more and more frustrated the more it happens.

AMOS: It's a drag.

THERAPIST: And has this stuff become a problem to you in some way?

AMOS: I don't care.

THERAPIST: Yeah, maybe you've figured out a way not to care, but has it become a problem to you?

AMOS: Nah.

THERAPIST: How about at home?

AMOS: Well, yeah.

THERAPIST: How so?

AMOS: My [foster] parents get all bent out of shape when the principal calls, or if I get suspended and I have to stay at home alone. They hate that.

THERAPIST: So they get concerned when the principal calls?

AMOS: They take their side. They all gang up on me then.

THERAPIST: So you feel like it's just you against all these grownups. That's the pits.

AMOS: I don't care. That's just the way it is. I just gotta watch out for *numero uno.*

THERAPIST: Hey, Spanish. I speak Spanish.

AMOS: My best friend is Ricardo. He's half black, half Puerto Rican. He's taught me lots of words, like *pendejo, hijo de puta . . .*

THERAPIST: Oh, that's okay, I get the message. Those were words I wasn't even allowed to hear when I was a kid, much less say them . . .

AMOS: (*Laughing*) I got some other ones too . . .

THERAPIST: Nah, nah, that's okay. Hey, listen, Amos, would it be okay with you if I asked your foster parents to come in so we could all figure out how to help you get this teacher off your back?

AMOS: What? Yeah, I guess so. But they're not gonna listen to me when I talk . . . they think they know everything, but they don't.

THERAPIST: Sometimes parents just get too worried about their kids. Sometimes that stops them from listening to the whole story.

AMOS: Yeah, my side.

THERAPIST: Yeah, and I think that would be important, so we can figure out how to help you with your feeling picked on and pissed off at school.

AMOS: Yeah, okay.

THERAPIST: But I also heard from your social worker that even if you don't like your teacher this year, your grades have been really good.

AMOS: I guess.

THERAPIST: You guess? She said your last report card had two A's.

AMOS: Yeah, and a D.

THERAPIST: And here I am picking on the good stuff, and you're only noticing the bad.

AMOS: Well, I can do better.

THERAPIST: I'm sure you can.

As this excerpt indicates, when I listened to Amos and was sympathetic to his side of things, he became more receptive. My leverage appeared to be with his concerned foster family. Once he identified that his behavior at school was a problem, in that his foster parents had to be notified and then they became worried and increased their monitoring of him, I knew I had something that we could work on.

The family sessions were productive. Amos had been correct

in that his foster parents did not want to listen to his side of things, and even accused him of lying. However, when I asked him to role play with me how the teacher scolded him in public, they seemed alarmed that the teacher would use the language she did and be so globally condemning of a young man they loved very much.

The principal had told the social worker during the referral that this was the first year that Amos had been a problem in the classroom, and that there was an option to move him to another teacher's class. Amos opted to stay in the first teacher's class, and much later in treatment confided to me that this teacher physically resembled his mother. Apparently the fact that she reminded him of his mother caused a range of emotions for him, and eventually he confided that he acted "extra rowdy" in her presence—perhaps wanting her attention, even if it was negative.

I worked with Amos for 9 months, and he was truly remarkable in how open and insightful he could be. During this time, his foster parents broke the news to him that they would become his adoptive parents. Even though Amos had a very strong negative reaction at first, insisting that he wanted to be on his own as soon as possible, after 2 or 3 weeks he began accepting the notion that he would not see his mother again. I thought it interesting that one of his first questions was, "Does that mean that I won't have to see my grandmother again, neither?" perhaps suggesting less disguised feelings about his sexual abuse.

When Amos was 16, he asked to see me when he got his girlfriend pregnant. Amos had dated the same girl for 2 years and felt strongly about marrying her in the future. However, he felt himself to be in acute crisis because he wasn't sure he was ready to be a father; he referred to his mother's difficulties in being such a young mother. At his request we had a meeting with his parents, his 15-year-old girlfriend, and the girl's parents. Amazingly, Amos was able to relate his concerns and fears to both sets of parents, and a joint decision was made to have a safe abortion. Five years later, I received a birth announcement for Amos's first child, a girl named Luz (the Spanish word for "light").

INVITING YOUNGSTERS TO SAY
WHAT THEY WANT

Another strategy for addressing resistance is to communicate that young clients are in control of what they say in therapy. I always tell them early on, "You can say as much or as little as you want in here," and "You'll be the judge of when you feel comfortable enough to say whatever you want."

I also tell kids, "Tell me what you think I need to know about you," conveying my respect for their ability to report the truth from their perspective. This segment illustrates how difficult it can be for adolescents to speak for themselves.

THERAPIST: So your parents called and told me there were some problems at home. How about if you tell me what you think I need to know?

ADOLESCENT: They must have told you.

THERAPIST: All they said was that there were problems.

ADOLESCENT: They think everything is my fault.

THERAPIST: They didn't say that to me.

ADOLESCENT: Well, that's what they holler to me all the time.

THERAPIST: What do you see as the problem?

ADOLESCENT: They think I'm using [drugs] all the time, but I'm not.

THERAPIST: Okay, so they think you're using, and that's a problem to them. How do you feel about it?

ADOLESCENT: I used to do drugs. I'm clean now. They don't believe me – they spy on me all the time. They go through all my stuff and my pockets and stuff, looking all the time.

THERAPIST: So what do you think is the problem?

ADOLESCENT: They say I act weird, but I think they act weird.

THERAPIST: What do you do that they think is weird?

ADOLESCENT: They say I don't talk to them and stuff. But I can't talk to them about stuff because they don't listen.

THERAPIST: And if they did listen, what would you want them to hear?

ADOLESCENT: That I'm not doing drugs any more.

THERAPIST: And what do you want me to know about you?

ADOLESCENT: They're on my back all the time.

THERAPIST: And how does that affect you?

ADOLESCENT: It feels like pressure, like they don't trust me.

THERAPIST: And how does that make you feel?

ADOLESCENT: Like they say, I feel like being in my room all the time, so they don't look at me funny.

THERAPIST: So you think they're always watching you, waiting for you to show signs of being on drugs or something?

ADOLESCENT: Yeah, but I'm not doing that any more, and they don't believe me.

THERAPIST: Why do you think they don't believe you?

ADOLESCENT: I don't know. Maybe, I don't know.

THERAPIST: What?

ADOLESCENT: Because my sister used to do drugs, and she stopped for a while, but she went back and OD'd.

THERAPIST: Your sister died?

ADOLESCENT: No, but she almost did, and now she lives in a drug center program in Colorado.

THERAPIST: I see. So your parents might worry that you'll go back and do drugs, and then something bad might happen to you.

ADOLESCENT: Yeah, I guess, but it messes my mind when they're weird all the time.

THERAPIST: So what would you want me to tell your parents if they listened to me?

ADOLESCENT: That they're not helping me out. They're making it worse.

THERAPIST: I hear you loud and clear.

This excerpt shows that when I first asked this client to tell me what I needed to know, he could only focus on his parents' behaviors. As we continued to talk, he began to make clear the problem from his perspective: The way they were choosing to be concerned about him and help him with his drug use was not helping him; as a matter of fact, it appeared to be making things worse. Now that I was equipped with this information, it was possible for me to communicate with his parents. Family therapy sessions consisted of my facilitating family members listening to, and understanding, each other as well as coming up with alternative ways of communicating their mutual concerns and needs.

BEING POSITIVE

It often takes every bit of creative strength to be positive with some adolescent clients, who can be rude, hostile, or annoyingly passive and compliant. And yet it often disarms adolescents when a therapist maintains a positive attitude toward them.

ADOLESCENT: You look like a whore today with all that makeup.

THERAPIST: You are certainly observant. Tell me, what would you suggest?

ADOLESCENT: Don't wear that red lipstick and take those black lines off your eyes.

THERAPIST: Okay, that sounds like good advice – go to a lighter shade of lipstick and soften the lines. Where did you learn so much about makeup?

ADOLESCENT: I know what looks good.

THERAPIST: Well, I appreciate constructive criticism.

Here's another example:

THERAPIST: So I'm wondering if anyone would like to make a suggestion about what to do in group next week.

ADOLESCENT: Yeah, let's go to the zoo.

THERAPIST: And what would we do at the zoo?

ADOLESCENT: Look at the animals and watch them shit and stuff.

THERAPIST: So you believe going to the zoo would be helpful to us in learning about the digestive system. That's certainly a very concrete way to learn. Anyone else have a suggestion?

When working with a very disruptive and talkative youngster in group, I commented, "It never ceases to amaze me how many different ways you have to keep everyone's attention focused on you. You are very resourceful the way you get that to happen." To another child who talked incessantly, I said, "I'm very impressed by how effectively you keep your mind and your mouth busy, because I think if suddenly you stop thinking and talking, you might have some difficult emotions come up." I paused myself, and then continued, "Some day you might want to experiment with taking little pauses, nothing too big, just to get used to the idea that you'll be able to stand the emotions that do come up."

To a child who farted in group therapy when he wanted to distract people, I said, "You know, it's not everyone who knows how to change the topic of conversation as quickly as you do. And although you've done it effectively by farting, next time I'd like you to expand your repertoire and ask to change the topic with words rather than farts."

NOT CHALLENGING INITIAL STATEMENTS

When kids say they don't care, that they don't feel anything, or that everything is fine, a therapist should not fall into the trap of challenging what they are saying. Instead, the therapist should inquire further, as in this example:

THERAPIST: So how were things with you this week?

ADOLESCENT: Fine.

THERAPIST: Ah . . . how so?

ADOLESCENT: What? It was fine.

THERAPIST: What was fine about your week?

ADOLESCENT: Nothing.

THERAPIST: Now I'm confused. Were things fine or not?

ADOLESCENT: Yeah, fine.

THERAPIST: I see. (*Silence*)

ADOLESCENT: What???

THERAPIST: Nothing.

ADOLESCENT: Why aren't you saying anything?

THERAPIST: Nothing for me to say.

ADOLESCENT: My mom is on a trip this week.

THERAPIST: Oh.

ADOLESCENT: My dad's been coming home earlier at night.

THERAPIST: How's that for you?

ADOLESCENT: Cool. It's cool to see him other than in the morning.

THERAPIST: What kinds of things are you men doing?

ADOLESCENT: We went to a movie, out for pizza, watched the game, stuff like that.

THERAPIST: Where's your brother?

ADOLESCENT: He went to my grandmother's . . . Mom still doesn't want him spending too much time alone with me.

THERAPIST: How does that make you feel?

ADOLESCENT: It's cool. I know why.

This was an adolescent who had sexually abused his younger brother, and the two boys were kept apart whenever possible. Both parents had been very angry at this adolescent, and trust was just beginning to be repaired.

DECODING AND SUPPORTING
THE INTENT OF THE SYMPTOM

As mentioned earlier, I try to find ways to support the intent of an adolescent's behavior without reinforcing negative ways of coping. The following excerpt is from a session with a 14-year-old European-American girl who had been sexually abused by her father for a full year. Not coincidentally, she had developed bulimia nervosa.

THERAPIST: Jane, when was the last time you binged and purged?

JANE: After dinner last night.

THERAPIST: Okay, let's spend some time on that specific time. What time was dinner served?

JANE: About 6:30.

THERAPIST: Okay, and what were you doing about 5 P.M.?

JANE: Just in my room, finishing up French homework, listening to music.

THERAPIST: How were you feeling?

JANE: Okay. A little tired because I had been running after school.

THERAPIST: Oh, that's right, and did you keep it down to 2 miles?

JANE: Yep, just under 2 miles.

THERAPIST: Okay, so you felt a little tired physically. How about emotionally?

JANE: I guess okay.

THERAPIST: You guess?

JANE: It was a pretty good day. I got a paper back with a good grade, and I didn't see those girls today.

THERAPIST: Oh, the ones that tease you?

JANE: Yeah, they weren't around today that I saw.

THERAPIST: Okay, so you're hanging out in your room. What else is going on in your house?

JANE: I can hear Mom and Lucy downstairs, banging things, you know, cooking.

THERAPIST: Anything else you notice?

JANE: Just the garlic smell . . . Lucy puts garlic in everything. I think she fries garlic every day.

THERAPIST: How do you like that smell?

JANE: Yummy.

THERAPIST: And what else is going on?

JANE: Nothing much. Lucy's jabbering, the phone's ringing, stuff like that.

THERAPIST: And you're still feeling relaxed?

JANE: Yeah.

THERAPIST: And then?

JANE: Mom calls me to dinner, so I go downstairs.

THERAPIST: You stop what you're doing and go down for dinner?

JANE: Yeah, and I say hi to Lucy and we sit down and everything looks pretty good. There's gobs of French fries, my favorite, and Mom is starting to parcel out the food.

THERAPIST: And how do you feel?

JANE: Mostly okay, but a little, you know – I know she's going to put just a little food on my plate. She's always nervous that I'm gonna throw up if I eat too much.

THERAPIST: And do you tell your mom anything?

JANE: No . . . I just don't want to make things worse. It's okay if she doles out the food . . . Oh yeah, then the phone rang, and it was for my father – one of his business people who doesn't know he doesn't live with us any more, so right away Lucy looks uptight, and my mom looks embarrassed, and you know, that's how it is.

THERAPIST: I see. So stuff that comes up about your dad still feels uncomfortable for everybody.

JANE: Yeah. Everybody gets really quiet, and Mom goes to the kitchen supposedly to get ketchup or something, but really just to wipe her eyes because there's already ketchup on the table.

THERAPIST: I see. So your mom gets weepy and you girls get quiet.

JANE: Yeah, but that's just the way it goes, I think everybody knows that now. I don't feel bad that I told on him, but I do feel bad for my mom. I think every now and then she just forgets what happened.

THERAPIST: And how does that make you feel?

JANE: Well, I know she just does that to feel better. I feel better when I pretend it didn't happen.

THERAPIST: Pretending doesn't always work too long, does it?

JANE: Nah.

THERAPIST: So now what happens?

JANE: It's really quiet, and Mom just looks down and eats, and then Lucy talks about what happened in her classes, and Mom pretends to be interested.

THERAPIST: And what do you do?

JANE: I just eat.

THERAPIST: You just eat?

JANE: Yeah, and that's when that funny thing happens when I feel like I'm not me any more, and I can see my fork picking up food and putting it into my mouth, but it's like my mouth isn't connected to my face, and I feel kind of numb.

THERAPIST: And this happened while your sister talked and your mother pretended to watch her?

JANE: Yeah, and then I'm in my little world, and I can't follow the conversation, and I'm just eating and eating, and taking more and more from the bowls.

THERAPIST: And do you feel any feelings?

JANE: No . . . just like I'm suspended . . . I can't explain it, like I'm not really there.

THERAPIST: I think you're explaining it really well. What do you know about how that feeling stops?

JANE: Last night I just know that my mom was grabbing a bowl from my hand and it was like a tug of war, and then I looked at her and sort of snapped out of it.

THERAPIST: So when you came back to the table you were fighting for the bowl?

JANE: Yeah.

THERAPIST: And how did your mom look?

JANE: Oh, she was pretty miffed, I think. Her eyeballs were glued on me.

THERAPIST: And what happened then?

JANE: I asked if I could be excused.

THERAPIST: And what did Mom say?

JANE: She said no, that I had to do the dishes.

THERAPIST: And . . . ?

JANE: That's what I did.

THERAPIST: How was that for you? It's been kind of a problem in the past.

JANE: I did okay until it came to the fries. Then I ate all the ones Lucy didn't, 'cause she's on a diet.

THERAPIST: And you washed the dishes without your mom being around?

JANE: Yeah, she got a phone call from Kim's mom.

THERAPIST: I see.

JANE: Yeah. Otherwise she would have been gawking at me, making sure I didn't eat everything.

THERAPIST: And what happened after dinner?

JANE: I finished the dishes quick, and while Mom was still on the phone I went up and barfed.

THERAPIST: You went to the bathroom and barfed?

JANE: No, Lucy was in there. They do that now – they spend time in the bathroom so I don't go barf.

THERAPIST: So where did you barf?

JANE: I had a plastic trash bag, and I barfed in that.

THERAPIST: And how did you feel after barfing?

JANE: Mostly okay.

THERAPIST: And what about the other parts?

JANE: Huh?

THERAPIST: You said "mostly" okay . . .

JANE: Oh, yeah. Well, you know, I felt kind of good and kind of bad.

THERAPIST: What felt good?

JANE: To get that stuff out of me, to clean myself out.

THERAPIST: Describe feeling good.

JANE: Relieved, sort of empty.

THERAPIST: Were you hungry?

JANE: Uh-uh.

THERAPIST: And what was the bad part?

JANE: Well, it's a little embarrassing to be gross like this.

THERAPIST: What do you mean?

JANE: Well, barfing all the time is kind of gross.

THERAPIST: Gross to who?

JANE: Well, to everybody.

THERAPIST: Does that include you?

JANE: Well . . .

THERAPIST: Well?

JANE: I know it's bad for me and everything, and I want to stop, but there's something about it . . .

THERAPIST: Something that makes you feel what?

JANE: I don't know. Bigger somehow.

THERAPIST: See if you can describe that more.

JANE: Well, like I'm in charge.

THERAPIST: What do you mean? What are you in charge of?

JANE: How much I eat.

THERAPIST: And how is that different than picking out the amount that you want to eat?

JANE: Because . . .

THERAPIST: Keep going . . .

JANE: Well, it's like I decide what stays inside me . . .

THERAPIST: And when couldn't you decide that?

JANE: What do you mean?

THERAPIST: Was there a time when something went inside you and you couldn't get it out?

JANE: Oooohhh, that's a gross thought.

THERAPIST: What?

JANE: I just remembered that when my dad stuck his dick inside me, I used to bear down really tight so that it wouldn't get in.

THERAPIST: Did it work?

JANE: Sometimes, but then he started using that jelly stuff, and then it didn't work so well.

THERAPIST: So you tried to keep his penis from coming inside you.

JANE: Hell, yes. Gross.

THERAPIST: And sometimes it worked and sometimes it didn't.

JANE: Yeah.

THERAPIST: And it sounds like now you do this thing with food where you decide what goes in and what comes out, and you feel more in charge.

JANE: Yeah. Weird, huh?

THERAPIST: Not so weird. Not so weird at all that you want to be in charge of your body. I think being in charge of what happens to your body is important to all of us. And especially if someone has done something to your body, or put something inside it, that you didn't like.

JANE: Yeah . . .

THERAPIST: And I think you've come up with a really good idea so far, and now my job is to help you come up with other ways that you can be in charge of your body that work just as well as eating and purging.

In this case example, Jane found a sense of empowerment from stuffing her body until it was full, and then depleting it. It's possible that this urge was propelled by a need to compensate for the sense of helplessness she felt in the face of sexual abuse – that is, her father stuffing her vaginal cavity and her inability to keep him out. It is also possible that the tension she perceived at the dinner table elicited her desire to quell her anxiety by overeating. If so, these two factors might have become interactive.

I chose this case example to illustrate that it is possible to support the intent of a symptom ("you've come up with a really good idea so far"), while at the same time encouraging the development of other, less damaging ways of coping. Eventually, Jane came up with an interesting solution: She asked her mother to take her back to ballet classes, which she had first taken as a very young child. She decided that she wanted to learn ballet so that she could move her body in very precise ways; she also wanted to develop muscles in her arms and thighs. There was a risk that she would undertake a rigorous dancing schedule with the same extreme intensity with which she pursued eating and purging. However, as we continued to work on Jane's sexual abuse, her family's reactions to her disclosure, and her preoccupation with her mother's mental health, her interests broadened beyond ballet as her social life became more active. (Her father had restricted her social contacts, preferring to keep her close to home and at his disposal.)

Two years after therapy was terminated, Jane called me to tell me that her sister, Lucy, had disclosed that she too had been sexually abused by their father. Lucy had also revealed that she felt tremendous guilt over her failure to disclose her abuse earlier. At the time it was happening, she threatened to tell her mother if her father did not stop abusing her. Although the abuse stopped without Lucy's telling her mother (and in that way her threat was effective), Lucy soon began suspecting on some level that her father was now abusing Jane. When Jane made her disclosure, Lucy was both "surprised and not surprised," and she concealed great remorse for having worried only about herself and her own protection. On the phone with me, Jane sounded concerned as she reported that Lucy had made a suicide attempt in college and "spilled the beans" on the psychiatric ward. Jane continued to be worried about her mother, but was relieved that the focus was no longer strictly on her. "Maybe now," Jane said, "Mom will accept once and for all that this really did happen." I saw Jane, her mother, and Lucy for 6 months of family therapy, and Lucy's therapist joined me as cotherapist. Finally, I worked with Jane's mother for approximately 2 years as she rebuilt her life—strengthening her relationship with her daughters, choosing and developing a career, dating, and purchasing a new home.

DOING INDIRECT RATHER THAN DIRECT WORK INITIALLY

Although I believe that at some point in time it is useful for many traumatized adolescents to process the traumatic events in a structured and focused way, not all adolescents respond to direct inquiry, and not all of them are able to engage with content material directly. For some adolescents who are reluctant and overwhelmed, it may be possible to work less directly and accomplish a great deal nevertheless. Here are a few ideas for "less direct" work:

1. Showing a videotape of adolescents talking about their lives. Two useful tapes are *Don't Get Stuck There,* from Boy's Town Press (1985), and *A Time to Tell,* from Walt Disney Educational Productions (1985).

2. Cutting out newspaper reports of events that occur in the lives of adolescents, and bringing them in for group or individual discussion.

3. Creating a mythical client who has the same problems, worries, or fears that the actual client has. The mythical client should be of the same gender and age as the real one. Often I'll give a mythical client a name that sounds like, or begins with the same letter as, the real client's name. Amazingly, adolescents are very receptive to identifying with the mythical client. I have never forgotten the following interaction with a 16-year-old Hispanic adolescent who had been forcibly sodomized by his uncle. I used this intervention after 3 months of sessions in which hardly a word was spoken between us. Up to that time I had tried talking myself; asked him to draw; watched videos with him; offered him the opportunity to make a sandtray (he declined); asked him to communicate with me through letter; and been completely quiet myself, telling him that this was his time and he needed to help me understand what he wanted to work on.

THERAPIST: (*Looking very worried*) Wow. You won't believe the kid I just saw.

CLIENT: (*No response*)

THERAPIST: No one will believe me when I tell them about this kid.

CLIENT: (*No response*)

THERAPIST: I don't think I've ever seen anything quite like it, and I've been working with kids a long time.

CLIENT: (*Making eye contact*) What?

THERAPIST: I don't know if I can talk to you about it. I'm not sure I even understand it myself. Wow. I just don't get it at all.

CLIENT: What?

THERAPIST: I just saw this kid. I've never seen anyone quite like him. He was unbelievable.

CLIENT: Why?

THERAPIST: Well, let me back up. Let's see what I can tell you to describe this situation. (*Hesitating*) It's just that he was so unusual . . .

CLIENT: Just tell me.

THERAPIST: His name is Simón.

CLIENT: Simón? (*Pronouncing it correctly*)

THERAPIST: Yeah, Simón.

CLIENT: Where's he from?

THERAPIST: Somewhere in Central America . . . Where are you from?

CLIENT: Nicaragua.

THERAPIST: He might be from there. Maybe El Salvador, I'm not sure.

CLIENT: Yeah, so . . . ?

THERAPIST: He's almost 17.

CLIENT: Yeah.

THERAPIST: Well, he had something really bad happen to him.

CLIENT: What, he was raped too?

THERAPIST: How did you guess?

CLIENT: You told me you talk to kids who get raped all the time.

THERAPIST: Well, yeah, he got raped too.

CLIENT: Yeah, so . . . ?

THERAPIST: Well, he just kept his eyes closed the whole time, and he held his face in his hands.

CLIENT: He probably doesn't want you to see him.

THERAPIST: Really? Is that it? Why not? What would I see?

CLIENT: You're a woman. You don't get it. For a guy, this is a whole different thing. The guy is probably afraid that anyone will see him now. [This youngster was identifying with the stigmatization and shame of sexual abuse for male children.]

THERAPIST: But why? It's not his fault.

CLIENT: He don't know that. Just 'cause you say it doesn't make it so, you know.

THERAPIST: So you think he might feel like he did something wrong.

CLIENT: Yeah, like he shouldn't have let it happen.

THERAPIST: But he got overpowered by a grownup.

CLIENT: Don't matter. He might think he should have protected himself.

THERAPIST: Wow, that's tough. I don't know how to get him to bring his hands down from his face.

CLIENT: Let him alone.

THERAPIST: What do you mean?

CLIENT: Let him keep his hands up. He don't want to show his face anywhere yet. He'll be okay later.

THERAPIST: You really think so?

CLIENT: Yeah . . . (*Shifting his weight*) He's gotta get to know you first.

As this excerpt indicates, this adolescent was able to be empathetic to my mythical client but not to himself. At the same time, this mythical client helped and allowed me to get to know my own client better. Interestingly, the actual client would ask about the mythical one at each session, tell me what to tell him, and suggest questions I should ask or statements I should make, each revealing his own deepest thoughts, fears, and worries.

DISCUSSING PROBLEMS IN GENERIC FASHION

Another helpful approach is to talk about adolescents with specific problems in generic fashion. For example, when working with adolescents who have been victimized, I often ask the following questions—not in any particular order or at any particular time, but scattered throughout our sessions. These questions may be similarly addressed in group meetings:

Why do you think people abuse children?
What kind of people abuse children?
What kind of children do they pick to abuse?
What do they say to themselves about what they're doing?
How do people who abuse children get caught?
What should happen to people who abuse children?
What kind of lessons do they need to be taught?
How do children who get abused feel?
What kinds of thoughts worry them or confuse them?
What kinds of problems do abused children have?
What helps children who are abused?
Who are some of the people abused children can talk to?

This type of generic talk allows young clients to bring out their concerns in a safe way. Talking about others affords the distance that many clients prefer.

USING "AS IF" INTERVENTIONS

An "as if" intervention invites an adolescent to talk about something in a manner that is one step removed from giving personal details. Notice how effective this is in the following example:

CLIENT: I don't want to talk about it.

THERAPIST: What will happen if you did talk about it?

CLIENT: I'd probably feel worse.

THERAPIST: And let's imagine you did talk about it, and you did feel worse. What would you feel worse about?

CLIENT: Because it makes me feel like I did something wrong.

THERAPIST: And if you did something wrong, what would that have been?

CLIENT: You know, when I took the money.

THERAPIST: Okay, and let's say you took the money. What was there to feel bad about?

CLIENT: 'Cause I should have said not at that point.

THERAPIST: And if you would have said no, then how would you feel?

CLIENT: Better about myself.

THERAPIST: Because?

CLIENT: Because I wouldn't have got a reward for what I did.

THERAPIST: And let's say you did it to get the reward?

CLIENT: Well, I didn't.

THERAPIST: But if you did, then what?

CLIENT: Well, I don't know.

THERAPIST: Would that make you a bad person?

CLIENT: No, not really.

THERAPIST: Would that make you a better person?

CLIENT: No.

THERAPIST: What would it make you?

CLIENT: A scaredy cat.

THERAPIST: So you might have felt scared to not take the money.

CLIENT: Yeah. Scared. And I didn't spend the money either.

BEING RESPECTFUL AND MAINTAINING CLEAR BOUNDARIES

Sometimes adolescents can provoke negative responses in adults by using provocative language or behavior. Such provocations in therapy may elicit a broad range of countertransferential response, including punitive, nurturing, overprotective, overfunctioning, or erotic reactions. It is critical for therapists to keep calm, and approach adolescents with the same respect they would afford adults. At the same time, setting limits and maintaining clear boundaries are vitally important to the therapeutic relationship.

Adolescents often relate to clinicians as if they were extensions of their parents (i.e., authority figures with control over their lives), or they may try to "buddy up" in order to loosen perceived controls. Particularly with adolescents, clinicians need to behave responsibly—discouraging too-familiar behaviors, inappropriate sexualization, or aggressive (or passive–aggressive) behaviors. Unacceptable behaviors must be explicitly described as such; firm limits must be set; and alternative behaviors must be suggested.

As an example, I once worked with a highly sexualized youngster who utilized her sexuality whenever she wanted somethng done for her, or wanted something done in a particular manner. I remember saying to her, "When you bat your eyelashes, move your eyebrows up and down, lower your tone of voice, and start rubbing your thighs, you are presenting yourself in a sexualized way. Acting this way won't work for you with me, so it would be more useful if you verbalized what you want right now, or found some more useful way to somehow let me know what it is you want." It would have been insufficient to say, "You're being seductive," or some such abstract description of what the youngster was doing. Some clinicians keep these observations to themselves, or document them in their notes without addressing the behavior directly; however, I think that direct attention to such behavior is the most useful response.

AVOIDING POWER STRUGGLES

One of the most important principles in working with adolescents is to avoid power struggles at all costs. Therapists who give adolescent clients as much choice as possible—who let them select topics for discussion, times of appointments, and ways in which they may communicate—usually will have greater success in building rapport.

It hardly ever works to try to "be right" in therapy with adolescents. If it is important for them to keep something private, or to assert a particular explanation or excuse, they should be allowed to do that until they no longer need to do so. This is especially true if adolescents insist that prior abuse meant nothing, wasn't important, or didn't affect them. I usually tell clients that I hear what they're saying at this particular moment, that they may feel differently at different times, and that I'll probably bring the topic up again from time to time. Denial is a useful defense, and the best approach to it mixes patience with perserverance. It is never helpful to avoid all painful or difficult material, simply because the adolescent persists in denying content or impact; doing so colludes with denial and can reinforce the adolescent's belief that the material cannot be adequately addressed.

A related rule of thumb has to do with disengaging from hostile interactions with adolescents, even when the provocations may be intense. The responses to such provocations can escalate, perpetuate, or help to resolve particular interactions, and clinicians have an opportunity and a responsibility to role-model appropriate behaviors.

BEING CREATIVE AND DYNAMIC

I find that there is a fine line between working "too hard" on the one hand, and making sure that I am sufficiently prepared with plans and alternative plans to engage and maintain the interest of adolescents (who are often easily bored) on the other. In this age of interactive media, youngsters are often used to, and require, a high level of activity to sustain their attention.

Luckily, clinicians have a range of creative resources available; a number of authors continue to document creative strategies that promote therapeutic goals. Therapists should be familiar with the literature so that they don't have to reinvent the wheel, or find themselves frustrated when they run out of ideas. Three of the best books on working with adolescents I have found are those by Carrell (1993), Friedberg, Mason, and Fidaleo (1993), and Young, West, Smith, and

Morgan (1994). In addition, there are two books written specifically for abused adoelscents that I highly recommend (Bean & Bennett, 1993; Mather & Debye, 1994). And lastly, although Sonkin's
(1992) book was written primarily for men who were abused during childhood, I have used many of its concepts and suggestions with
abused adolescent males.

MAKING USE OF NONVERBAL
FORMS OF THERAPY

There are many compelling reasons to avoid overreliance on verbal
communication in therapy. First, adolescents may feel uncomfortable talking with adults in general and therapists in particular. Because of developmental issues, youngsters often feel "in between"
childhood and adulthood, and are usually more at ease with peers.
There is also the real possibility that therapists are seen as mind read-
ers of sorts and that adolescents may be afraid of self-disclosure. Fur-
thermore, some adolescents may have a "them–us" concept of
adult–adolescent relationships and may feel lack of trust for anyone
who is not a contemporary.

Second, as I have said throughout the book, the disclosure and
processing of abuse can feel burdensome and problematic to many
youngsters. Victims of violence and assault characteristically under-
report those crimes, particularly when they implicate friends, family members, lovers, or parents. This hesitency to make statements
about abuse often interferes with verbal therapy, and clinicians must
have a broader repertoire of strategies to implement.

Over the years I have had great success using (or referring my
clients to use) a variety of expressive therapies, such as art therapy,
collage making, clay sculpture, sandworld or sandplay therapy, music
or movement therapy, drama, pantomine, and the making of film
or video documentaries. So much did I value these strategies that
in 1994 I became a full-time student in George Washington University's art therapy program, so that I could futher explore the depths
of opportunity available through creative therapy.

At this point in my training and supervision, I cannot say enough about how ample the theory and practice of art therapy are, and how much I've learned about art therapy's curative elements. I wish I had been able to pursue this study much earlier, and although I am grateful that I used art work in my therapy with great caution in the past, I am extremely grateful to learn the broad implications of its use. Art therapy is a type of intervention with the potential to produce great insight, growth, and change in clients. At the same time, in the hands of untrained clinicians, art work can produce flooding and/or nontherapeutic regression instead of empowerment and useful change. I therefore encourage clinicians to become well informed and trained about the expressive therapies prior to incorporating them into their work, because these are very powerful tools that must be properly understood and implemented if they are to be of true service to the clients.

The field of art therapy has been evolving since the 1920s, and a substantial literature has been compiled. There are a number of basic texts that will introduce the reader to the foundations of art therapy for children and adults (see, e.g., Naumburg, 1987; Rubin, 1984, 1987; Ulman & Dachinger, 1975; Kramer, 1971). There are also several excellent journals devoted to research and clinical material on art therapy: the *American Journal of Art Therapy, The Arts in Psychotherapy, Art Therapy: Journal of the American Art Therapy Association,* and the *Journal of Multicultural and Cross-Cultural Research in Art Education.*[1] Lastly, for purposes of the present book, Linesch's (1988) book aptly explains the many uses of art therapy in the assessment and treatment of adolescents.

WORKING "IN CONTEXT"

Children and adolescents who are brought for therapy bring their unique realities, or context. Some youths have compelling struggles

[1]The journals can be obtained from the following addresses: *American Journal of Art Therapy,* Vermont College of Norwich University, Montpelier, VT 05602; *The Arts in Psychotherapy,* Pergamon Press, Maxwell House, Fairview Park, Elmsford, NY

as a result of racism, sexism, poverty, unemployment, or other demanding social circumstances. More and more, I am working with youth for whom violence is a daily reality, and for whom the dangers of prostitution, car theft, or forging checks are secondary to the dangers of hunger, lack of shelter, or despair. It is unreasonable to focus therapy on superficial problems such as communication, or poor school grades, when parents and children suffer a perilous existence. Our clinical interventions must be provided in context, so they make sense to the families we seek to serve, and so they aggressively pursue necessary resources. The narrow definition of "therapist" needs to be broadened to include the concept of advocacy and provision of concrete services. In order to be effective advocates, we must interact with our communities; give voice to our concerns through policies and legislation; and commit a percentage of our time, however we see fit, to social and political concerns.

CONCLUSIONS

In short, working with adolescents is both challenging and rewarding, and requires careful navigation to avoid obstacles that can interfere with the formation of a solid therapeutic relationship with its inherent potential benefits. Because adolescents often have mixed feelings about adults in position of authority, clinicians must take extraordinary efforts to establish themselves as trustworthy, and create a safe and appropriate therapy context in which adolescents feel that the clinicians care for them, respect them, and are trying to help them maximize their own potential for growth and health.

Clear boundaries are critical to advance therapy goals. I have observed one therapeutic error with great frequency: therapists' efforts to befriend adolescents by acting "cool" and being uncharacteris-

10523; *Art Therapy: Journal of the American Therapy Association,* 1202 Allanson Road, Mundelein, IL 60060; *Journal of Multicultural and Cross-Cultural Research in Art Education,* Department of Art Education, School of Architecture and Allied Arts, University of Oregon, Eugene, OR 97403.

tically entertaining and relaxed. I recognize that therapists may attempt a more uninhibited approach in order to engage young clients in therapy, but often this approach is confusing at best and counterproductive at worst. Abused adolescents in particular may have had devastating experiences with either enmeshed or too-loose boundaries, and may seek clarity in relationships. Establishing appropriate clinical boundaries will also aid clinicians in the process of becoming trustworthy.

CHAPTER SEVEN

Treatment Modalities

I have provided illustrations of work with abused adolescents in individual and group therapy throughout the book. Both modalities are necessary and accomplish distinctive goals, but my experience has shown me that the best approach is to provide them sequentially if at all possible. Individual therapy accomplishes a number of specific goals, as discussed below; however, group therapy allows clinicians to observe their clients interacting with peers, and thus to assess the clients' social skills and their negotiation of relational issues (joining, initiating and responding to contact from others, etc.). In addition, other modalities (such as family therapy and pair therapy) promote the overriding goal of treatment: helping adolescents find ways to remove obstacles to their own development, including the obtainment of safe and consistent environments.

In other words, adolescents with histories of victimization have sustained emotional injuries that may affect their sense of identity, their future orientation, their feelings of safety, their ability to trust, and so forth. They may continue to live in environments that are unrewarding, non-nurturing, or nonprotective, and because of their age and the perception of others that their risk is now decreased, they may have to "make the best" of their situations. As clinicians, we are often in the position of having to fortify adolescents so that they may feel empowered to cope with the realities of their situation. We must reinforce their abilities to avoid or diffuse conflict, to protect and care for themselves, and to access internal and external support systems. As mentioned in the previous chapter, therapeutic efforts must be offered within each individual's context.

Therapists must function outside traditional therapy modes to access and mobilize community resources, funding sources, housing possibilities, and other types of concrete help for families who will be unable or unwilling to engage in traditional psychotherapy until physical safety issues are addressed. Different modalities of therapy allow us to do this in different ways.

INDIVIDUAL TREATMENT

Individual treatment appears particularly relevant for establishing therapy in a low-risk environment; modeling healthy relational interactions (and thus giving adolescents a more optimistic view of the potential in human relationships); helping adolescents perceive their therapists (and, by implication, the process of therapy) as trustworthy; addressing issues of identity and esteem in a context that is free from the stress of peers; and broaching sensitive, private matters that may elicit feelings of stigmatization, shame, or disloyalty. It takes time for most abused adolescents to develop comfort in the context of a therapeutic relationship, and individual therapy provides individualized attention and focus so that the therapeutic relationship develops more quickly.

At the same time, it is this very element of individual therapy—individualized attention and focus on the client—that may elicit severe anxiety in abused adolescents and may interfere with the development of a therapeutic relationship. Many abused adolescents cannot help viewing therapy as a high-risk activity: It's a one-on-one personal relationship with an authority figure, behind closed doors, ostensibly to discuss private matters in confidence. For many abused adolescents these dynamics may be very threatening, because they resemble the dynamics of situations in which people violated their trust in the past.

As I've discussed elsewhere (Gil, 1991), the lessons of child abuse are insidious and far-reaching. Among those lessons is one that affects trust of others. When children are hurt by people who say they love them, the message is quite clear: "People who love you hurt

you." Therefore, intimacy suggests threat. In therapeutic relationships, clinicians attempt to make adolescents feel respected and cared
for. If they succeed, adolescents who bring with them these heart-
felt lessons about the nature of relationships will feel anxious and
threatened, and will usually pull back by missing appointments or
acting in provocative ways. This internalized conflict about accepting versus rejecting positive attention continues to be activated
throughout the therapy process.

When clinicians find that their best efforts to engage adolescents
in individual therapy fail, the most natural reaction is to feel as if
therapy has failed altogether. In fact, an adolescent's inability to engage in individual therapy may suggest that a clinician has succeed-
ed in promoting a caring environment and now must help the
adolescent tolerate positive attention and regard.

One tactic that often helps is for clinicians to take a more neu-
tral stance with adolescents, making explicit what they have observed. For example, if an adolescent is resistant and nonverbal at
this point, I may say something like this:

> "I've noticed that you've been struggling to feel comfortable in
> our therapy sessions the last 2 weeks. I think that there's a lot
> going through your mind. Let me tell you what I think, and
> then you can tell me how close I get to the mark. I think that
> you have felt pretty positive about the work we've done in here,
> and how you are treated. I listen to you; I'm interested; I care
> about your feelings. This may not feel too comfortable to you
> because you're not used to it, or you may not trust it complete-
> ly. If I'm interested in you, or if I care how you're doing, you
> may think that the other shoe is going to drop—that is, that I'm
> going to change, and in some way hurt or betray you."

If an adolescent is recalcitrant but more verbal, I may ask directly
what's going on from his or her perspective. Making the problem
explicit in this way allows for fruitful discussion about the issues
that may be underlying resistance. However, if adolescents persist
in disengaging from the therapy process in individual treatment,
group therapy may be a realistic alternative.

GROUP THERAPY

Group therapy is a good means of obtaining a fuller view of an adolescent's functioning. Although I have mentioned earlier that I use individual and group therapy sequentially, a period of conjoint work can sometimes be compensatory: Issues that surface during group therapy can be processed during individual treatment.

Group therapy places adolescents within a system that is a microcosm of larger or more complex systems, such as family, school, or church. Many issues must be negotiated within the group, such as how to join, participate, maintain boundaries, utilize the experience, and make the experience safe. In addition, adolescents face an array of personalities, just as they do in their daily lives; they will gravitate toward some of these, and will reject or avoid others. How they manage relational demands, and what skills they employ to communicate their needs, become important data for clinicians.

Joining is particularly difficult. Many adolescents with histories of abuse expect rejection or ridicule from others. They feel "different," and as a result isolate themselves from others. For many adolescents joining groups for abused adolescents, the sense of being different will be challenged immediately as they learn that everyone in the group was abused as a child. Even after they learn this, however, some adolescents will begin to make distinctions about type or frequency of abuse, designed to maintain their sense of having problems unlike anyone else's. Often this sense of being "different" takes a great deal of time to recede. I have sometimes encountered youngsters who hold on to their sense of being "different," or of being abuse survivors, as a form of identity. As their sense of self expands beyond the experiences of victimization they have had in the past, their identities are more fully developed to embrace additional information about themselves.

Abused adolescents are often hypervigilant in groups, scanning the environment for signs of rejection. This necessary ability to protect themselves from perceived danger often deflects their energy from being receptive to positive interactions with the group. Clinicians must remain alert to the ways in which adolescent defenses can prevent positive contact with the environment.

For example, in many groups I've found one or two adolescents who habitually "space out" during group sessions when the going gets rough. When painful, emotional issues are discussed, these youngsters avail themselves of the ability to dissociate and remove themselves emotionally from the group experience. As a result, adolescents don't feel the discomfort or pain elicited by the group's discussion, but they also don't feel the relief and comfort of working through a difficult emotion and achieving resolution. When this happens, I make the process explicit by asking the dissociating adolescents what precipitated their response, and asking them to be present for a review of the discussion. Doing this normalizes the process of dissociation, asserting its positive value while at the same time acknowledging its disadvantages. Group discussions on the use of defensive strategies are always worthwhile.

Groups for abused adolescents also allow adolescents opportunities to tell their stories from their point of view, to accept feedback from others, to identify with both the problems and solutions of others, and to feel emotionally connected or affiliated to others. As I describe in more detail below, Selman and Schultz (1990) have documented the importance of friendships in childhood and adolescence, and groups can offer abused adolescents their first opportunities to reach out, accept, and be accepted by others.

Unfortunately, group therapy does not work for everyone. Some young clients are overstimulated and overwhelmed by groups and become disruptive, noncompliant, hostile, and threatening, or simply cannot, or do not, participate in the process. In these situations, pair therapy may be an option (see below). Donaldson and Cordes-Green (1994) have written a scholarly review of the assumptions made about group therapy, as well as its empirically supported benefits; they also provide a structured format for creating and implementing group therapy for adult incest survivors, which is useful information for clinicians conducting group therapy with abused adolescents.

PAIR THERAPY

I began doing "pair therapy" about 10 years ago with two female clients who were adult survivors of childhood abuse. I initiated the process of having these two clients meet together because they both desperately needed human contact with someone other than a therapist, and they were both fiercely afraid of interacting with others, barely leaving their homes except to go to work. Both had jobs that required (or allowed) them to be isolated – one as a toll collector, the other as a bus driver. Both jobs were interesting because they provided a service to members of the public but required minimal interactions with them.

Therapy sessions with these two unrelated women who had similar issues and concerns were very successful. They felt "connected" by the nature of their problems, and they felt relieved to find someone else who felt similar concerns. Slowly, they developed a warm and positive relationship in which they confided in each other, taking more and more controlled risks as time went by. They looked forward to coming to therapy, and the therapy process eventually took a back seat to the friendship that developed before me. Each client was delighted and validated by her newfound friendship – something each had longed for and found elusive. Finally, the two settled into a mutually beneficial relationship outside the therapy process. Both reported that having a friend had made it more possible for them to consider themselves "normal people" who were no longer petrified by human contact.

In 1991, I bought Selman and Schultz's book *Making a Friend in Youth: Developmental Theory and Pair Therapy.* I was thrilled to find that these authors had devoted significant time and scientific study to the therapeutic value of bringing together two clients (in their case, children) who could explore the concept of forming friendships in a therapeutic relationship. Their pioneering work in this area is essential reading, whether a clinician ever considers doing pair therapy or not. Pair therapy is certainly an option in working with adolescents who have been abused and who by definition have disturbed interpersonal interactions. It is possible to tap their innate capacities for relating to others by removing obstacles created by their earlier experiences.

FAMILY THERAPY

Family therapists have long considered adolescents' problems in the context of their families. Considerable attention has been given to the treatment of adolescents and their families, and I concur with the basic premises provided in much of the literature on family therapy with adolescents.

I do believe, however, that abused adolescents can present an additional challenge in such therapy, because a certain amount of damage has been done to the child's developmental process by the time the family enters treatment. As I have emphasized throughout this book, child abuse or neglect compromises a youngster's sense of identity, safety, and personal power. Initially, this youngster may not be able to participate fully in family therapy because of his or her feelings of vulnerability and learned helplessness. As a matter of fact, the experience of family therapy, unless the youngster has already established a relationship with a therapist/ally, may feel like another form of abuse – a context in which, once again, the adult's needs take precedence over the adolescent's.

I recommend making efforts to build a therapeutic relationship with an adolescent abuse survivor in individual therapy first. The adolescent needs an advocate, a trusted helper – someone who will "even the odds" in the context of a dysfunctional, abusive home. Without this foundation, the adolescent may not be able to embrace the potential benefits of family therapy. An abused adolescent may not have a strong enough voice to be heard over others; an individual therapist will listen to the adolescent first, learning the young person's story and assessing his or her needs, and then determine the most beneficial therapy format.

A systemic approach is always useful (Gil, 1995). However, in work with an abusive family, it may be more effective to meet with members separately, slowly rebuilding the family interactions piece by piece. Youngsters who have been abused or neglected are my first priority; they are my primary clients, and since I will always work in their best interests, their families inevitably become my clients as well. The best thing I can do to help troubled youths is to help ensure a safe environment – one that supports and encourages their growth and development. I cannot imagine a situation in which I would not offer family therapy when an adolescent has been abused. Of course the "family" may not be the biological family of the child; I may not have access to the biological family; or the family may refuse treatment. Therefore, I may do "family therapy" with the adolescent alone, or I may be working in conjoint sessions with the child's external family or family systems.

In the following excerpt, the adolescent client (15-year-old Robbie, who described himself as "half Irish, half French") was my focal point as issues of childhood abuse and neglect were discussed in a family therapy session concerning the adolescent's return home. This adolescent had been sexually abused by his older sister, and physically abused by his mother's boyfriend. The session included my client, Robbie; his mother; his sister, Sharon; and the mother's husband (formerly her abusive boyfriend), Stan.

ROBBIE: I'm not listening to what he says. I don't care if you're married. He's not my father.

MOTHER: I know he's not your father. Thank God he's not your father. But he is going to live with us.

ROBBIE: I'm not taking any bull off him any more.

MOTHER: You've got to give him a chance.

ROBBIE: Yeah, whatever.

THERAPIST: Robbie, there are some important things you want to say to Stan, your mom, and your sister today. I know it's hard for you to be clear with them, but I'd like you to take a minute, think about the main thing you want to make clear, and give it a shot.

ROBBIE: I'm not letting him put another finger on me again. I want him to know it's not going to be like it was before.

THERAPIST: You want it clear that he's not to hit you again.

ROBBIE: Yeah.

THERAPIST: Stan, is that clear to you?

STAN: Yeah, I know, I know. I don't need to hear this from him.

THERAPIST: Well, he needs to say it to you. It's important to him.

STAN: Yeah, well, I got some things to say too.

THERAPIST: That's fine, Stan. Everyone gets to talk in here. I just want to make sure that Robbie gets a chance because sometimes in the past he's had a hard time talking to you guys, and then he gets quiet and refuses to talk. And, Mrs. L., I'd like to hear what you think about Robbie's statement to Stan.

MOTHER: Well, I think he knows how I feel.

THERAPIST: Robbie, do you know how your mom feels?

ROBBIE: No.

THERAPIST: This is a good time . . . [requesting the mother talk to Robbie directly].

MOTHER: I've told you how sorry I was that I didn't help out more when you and Stan got into it. I don't know what else to say.

THERAPIST: What got in your way of helping out?

MOTHER: I just didn't think it would go so far.

ROBBIE: Mom, you were there lots of times when he was beating me up. Don't say you weren't.

MOTHER: I just didn't know what to do . . .

THERAPIST: What did you try?

MOTHER: Well, I did talk to Stan, once he calmed down. I kept asking him not to drink so much, because that's when he gets ornery and everything bothers him.

STAN: I haven't had a drink in 6 months now.

ROBBIE: Well, la di da.

THERAPIST: Stan, I think it's great that you've stopped drinking. It takes a lot of strength to make that commitment and stick to it. It's probably gonna take a while for Robbie to feel friendlier to you, or to be supportive. One of the things we'll continue to work on is your relationship. There's a lot of trust to be rebuilt again, and it may never work out too great. We'll have to wait and see. The best thing you can do is be consistent and keep your promises.

But back to you, Mrs. L. You were saying that you tried to help Rob by talking to Stan when he was sober. Anything else?

MOTHER: I tried to stop them sometimes.

ROBBIE: How'd you do that, Mom?

MOTHER: You remember, I tried to pull him off you once.

ROBBIE: Oh, yeah, once. Big deal.

THERAPIST: What would you have wanted your mom to do, Robbie?

ROBBIE: Kick him out of the house for hitting Sharon and me like he did.

THERAPIST: Mom, what do you think of that?

MOTHER: I'm just glad it's over, and it's not gonna happen any more.

THERAPIST: Is there anything you want to say to Robbie about what happened in the past?

MOTHER: Well, just that I'm sorry it happened.

THERAPIST: Robbie?

ROBBIE: I don't know. She just can't say "I'm sorry," and make it all better.

THERAPIST: Apologies don't seem enough.

ROBBIE: Nah, not for all the shit I went through. I still got scars to prove it.

THERAPIST: Scars inside and out, right, Robbie?

ROBBIE: (*No response*)

THERAPIST: Stan, how do you think the beatings affected Robbie?

STAN: I know it hurt him. I know.

THERAPIST: How do you know?

STAN: Shit, that's how it was with me. My dad beat the living daylights out of me when I was a kid.

THERAPIST: And what was that like for you?

STAN: Pretty shitty. I ran away at 14, got a job, never looked back.

THERAPIST: I see. So you got out of there as soon as you could. Never went back.

STAN: Nope. Never have gone back, either.

THERAPIST: That sounds rough. Running away that young tells me something about how hard it was for you, Stan.

MOTHER: I'm sure that's why he drank so much. Basically, he's a really good person.

ROBBIE: Oh right, Mom, he's a prince, and what am I?

MOTHER: Robbie, I love you, you're my son. You'll always be my son.

ROBBIE: But if it comes right down to it, you'll pick him, right?

MOTHER: No, honey. That's not right.

STAN: Your mother damn near kicked me out of your house, Robbie. She set down the rules. She wasn't gonna lose you.

MOTHER: Robbie, did you know that?

ROBBIE: Bull . . .

THERAPIST: Mrs. L., tell Robbie about the rules.

MOTHER: I told Stan that if he didn't sober up we wouldn't get married, and I wouldn't live with him.

THERAPIST: Tell Robbie about his coming home.

MOTHER: I made up my mind that we were going to get you back no matter what it took. I told Sharon, whatever had to happen with her therapy, or her moving out to college, and I told Stan. We are going to be a family again.

ROBBIE: Not as long as he's around.

MOTHER: I know it's going to be rough. I know you're really mad at Stan, and at me too because I stood by. But I'm gonna make it up to you, Robbie, you'll see.

THERAPIST: That's right, Robbie. Actions speak louder than words, and you're going to have to wait and see.

Sharon, you've been very quiet here today. Anything you want to add?

SHARON: I just feel really bad about what I did. When you talked about his scars, his inside scars, it made me think that I put some of those there too by making him do stuff with me (*crying a little, and using a soft voice*).

THERAPIST: Well, it's appropriate for you to feel some remorse, Sharon. What you did wasn't good to do, and it sounds like you've been thinking about that and working on it in therapy. And maybe now the important thing is to see what you can do to help Robbie.

SHARON: Yeah, I've already told him what I did was wrong.

THERAPIST: Robbie?

ROBBIE: What she did wasn't that bad. It didn't *hurt* me or anything.

THERAPIST: You don't see the molesting as something that was physically painful?

ROBBIE: No.

THERAPIST: Although you've had some other feelings about it, haven't you, Rob?

ROBBIE: I don't wanna talk about that now.

THERAPIST: Okay, maybe later–maybe sometime you, Sharon, and I should get together. You've gotta make sure you give her a chance to help you or make up to you what she's done. We can do that later.

SHARON: Yeah, I'd like to talk, just him and I.

THERAPIST: Sharon, how do you feel about your mother's wedding, and about Stan?

SHARON: I'm with Robbie about that. He's been really mean to us for a really long time, and I can't just forget like Mom did.

THERAPIST: Mom, have you forgotten?

MOTHER: Oh, no, those things are buried in my memory. Sometimes I dream about them. Sometimes I can see it, or hear it, like it was happening right now.

THERAPIST: I imagine the abuse is hard for everyone to forget.

STAN: I am gonna show these kids that I've changed, and I can take it if they are rude, or whatever they dish out. I'll just show them.

THERAPIST: As I've said, time will tell. What's important now is to try to make amends, try to have chances for everyone to heal and feel better. And . . . make sure it doesn't happen again. That's really important to Robbie, and it's really important to me that he be safe.

You know, Stan, you talked with a lot of sadness about how bad your beatings were, and how you ran away at 14. How you never wanted to go back. Probably afraid the same thing would happen, or convinced there was nothing back home for you. In a way, that's a little how I think Robbie feels. He sort of doesn't want to go home, doesn't trust that anything will be different, isn't sure what home will be like. You probably understand that better than any of us.

STAN: Yeah, I know that feeling.

THERAPIST: So it's gonna take a while for everyone to feel differently, and for trust to build up – trust that hasn't been there for a very long time.

STAN: Yeah. I know.

In this session, Robbie was my primary concern, although I related to other family members and empathized with their particular issues. My focus was on creating a safe enough environment for Robbie, and making sure that he knew what to do if he felt unsafe again.

There are many useful models of family therapy, and although a thorough review of these models is beyond the scope of this book, I will describe my own orientation. I consider myself primarily a structural family therapist who uses strategic approaches and is influenced by Bowenian, solution-focused, and narrative approaches.

Because abusive or neglectful families are usually multiproblem, dysfunctional families, I find Minuchin's (1974) structural family therapy to be a pivotal approach. The basic premise of structural family therapy is its emphasis on space configurations, such as closeness versus distance, inclusion versus exclusion, fluid versus rigid boundaries, and hierarchical arrangements regarding power and delegation of power. Minuchin (1974) notes how matching parts of a whole fit through a process called "complementarity." He also regards symptoms as fitting into dysfunctional configurations that may serve the developmental needs of the family. As opposed to focusing on the function of the symptom, structural therapy focuses on the organizational flaw reflected by the symptom. A structural therapist therefore engages in rebuilding efforts, designed to alter and (the therapist hopes) to improve the underlying structural problems in the family. Since abusive families are particularly susceptible to underlying structural problems (e.g., excessive closeness or distance) and boundary problems (i.e., either over- or underinvolvement of parents with their children), a structural approach is very useful.

Many therapists regard themselves as structural/strategic. Structural issues are often promoted by strategic approaches, which are most often problem-focused and brief, with an active therapist who often works in front of a one-way mirror. Strategic therapy was developed by Haley (1976) and Madanes (1981), and a basic premise is that pathology develops when there are confusions in existing hierarchies.

The Bowenian model also has relevance in working with abuse and neglect, since cross-generational transmission processes may exist with many abusive parents, who repeat their own histories of abuse. Bowen (1978) believed that it is impossible to see the nuclear family without viewing the broader context, the connection to the past. At the core of his theory is the process of differentiation of self–the individual's ability to maintain a degree of autonomy even when pressures for togetherness persist. In order for the individual to be autonomous, he must find his or her own identity, choices, sense of control, and instinct for the environment. Bowen proposed that therapists function not as therapists, but as "coaches," educators, or consultants.

In recent years, two other family therapy models have been developed and have enjoyed great popularity: solution-oriented and narrative therapy. Solution-focused therapy (O'Hanlon & Weiner-Davis, 1989) focuses on solutions rather than problems; suggests that symptoms do not serve functions; does not pursue the past, or origins of problems; and proposes that therapy can create change quickly (in four to five sessions, sometimes in one) by narrowing the discussion to solution-focused perspectives. Although I find this approach fascinating and congruent with my emphasis on not pathologizing and not labeling people, and I integrate it into my therapy approach whenever possible, I have not yet been able to execute the approach within the brief context that is suggested. Of course, it is possible that my own belief system regarding the need for careful construction of a safe therapeutic relationship, and the amount of time I believe this takes, interferes with my ability to carry out a pure solution-focused approach. I am still unwilling to discard some of the techniques, however – perhaps because I agree with O'Hanlon and Weiner-Davis's belief that "there is no one right theory of psychotherapy. Many different theories and many different techniques and approaches seem to produce change and positive results" (1989, p. 11). These authors add, "Instead of looking for the right theory of therapy, we should perhaps be searching in another direction . . . solutions rather than problems" (1989, p. 11), or successes in clinical practice rather than failures. Inevitably, all of us will repeat strategies that our clients find useful and discard those that do not produce effective change.

I have discussed narrative therapy in Chapter Four. I am more and more convinced of its applicability in cases of child abuse and neglect, particularly with individuals who have been victimized. This approach thoroughly respects the individual's internal resources, and encourages competency through rescripted narrations that shape expectations and realities.

SUMMARY AND CONCLUSIONS

In summary, a number of treatment modalities can be useful in work with abused adolescents. Friedrich (1995b) provides a thoughtful evaluation of how different treatment modalities address specific issues relating to attachment, dysregulation, and the self.

Because of abused adolescents' inherent problems, therapy may be a difficult process for them to participate in or trust. Careful efforts must be made to make therapy user-friendly, decrease both its apparent and its actual risks, and encourage youngsters to trust the therapeutic process itself. A combination of individual, group, and family work may be necessary to address issues of victimization, family support, and reunification. In addition, for adolescents with troubled interpersonal interactions, pair therapy may yield invaluable rewards.

Afterword

During a writing project, I find that particular clients and clinical situations come to the surface of my conscious awareness. I also notice that successful cases rise with positive associations, whereas cases that were difficult, or in which little change occurred, awaken feelings of trepidation and anxiety in me. Elsewhere (Gil, 1995), I have noted how much I've learned from both successes and failures, and how I've spoken of both at lectures but have been much more cautious about committing failures to the printed word. And yet the danger in writing exclusively about successful cases that achieved some positive resolution is that I may inadvertently give the impression that working with abused adolescents is easier than it might actually be, or that there is something unique about the way in which I conduct therapy. Neither statement is true.

Working with abused adolescents is tough–there are no two ways about it. These youngsters come to therapy with years and years of pain, feelings of helplessness, well-entrenched defenses, and enormous distrust of adults (and of human interactions in general). One of the hardest problems to contend with is their distrust. Sometimes young clients distrust me and other adults simply because we are adults, and I can't say I blame them one bit. The adults they have known so far have been unpredictable, unreliable, injurious, assaultive, detached, or critical. As a result, these adolescents become masters of disguise: They are often violent when they feel most helpless, sexual when they are most childlike or vulnerable.

For me, even more difficult than working with abused adolescents has been working with their families, who come weary, confused, disheartened, angry, despaired, and most of all skeptical that anything will help. In addition, parents may be simultaneously defensive and guilty, reluctant to discuss the past, and afraid that their parenting failures are all too apparent. If they have been abusive parents (and many of them have been), either they are self-righteous about their behavior, or they claim ignorance about the potential damage of their behavior. If they have neglected their children because of temporary incapacitation (caused by substance abuse, physical illnesses, domestic violence, or mental health problems), they may feel ashamed about their pasts. In either case, they exhibit behaviors parallel to those of their youngsters: They are well defended, distrustful, angry, and in great pain underneath it all.

For the most part, once I process my negative countertransferential responses, I have been able to find empathy for parents who too often have been ill prepared to be parents and may have been abused or neglected themselves. But there have been times when, try as I may, I have found it impossible to empathize with parents as they continue to exhibit total disregard for the youngsters in their care. Many of the children and adolescents I have worked with were not able to live with their original families, and it seemed everyone benefited from the youngsters' placement in a foster home, a group home, or a residential treatment center. I hoped that their transition into adulthood would be facilitated by their adult caretakers, and most of the time I was very impressed with the personnel in out-of-home-care facilities.

I want to emphasize the importance of staying aware of, and processing, the countertransference responses provoked by working both with abused adolescents and with their families. In particular, I have been mystified by how much my own adolescence passes before my eyes as I work with this population.

Mine was not the smoothest adolescence. I came to the United States from another culture (South America) at 14 years of age, leaving important friends and extended family at a time that was quite significant for young girls. I was approaching the age at which girls have their *Fiesta de Quinceañeras,* the South American equivalent of a coming-out party or debutante ball. I came kicking and screaming, since I felt that I was going to miss the most important transition of my life: I thought that the day after the party, I would somehow be transformed into a woman.

I mostly remember how excruciating it was that I did not fit in, had no friends, and was laughed at because I did not then speak correct English and because my name was different. In adolescence, everyone wants most of all to feel accepted and to belong to a group. As I tried to adjust or acculturate, my mother became anxious about the family's losing traditional values. I therefore experienced conflict and tension as a result of conflicting cultural demands. These experiences were painful; later, however, they allowed me as a therapist to connect with youngsters who presented with similar concerns. And yet I found it both advantageous and disadvantageous to have had these difficulties as a youngster.

Certainly I felt I could identify with some of my adolescent clients' feelings and defenses, and in that sense my experiences constituted an advantage. However, working with the youngsters' parents was more difficult and intense for me because of my own experiences. I found myself constantly self-evaluating, amazed at how many feelings this work provoked—feelings that I did not experience, for example, when working with younger children.

An interesting thing happened with my caseload: I work with abusive families, adult abuse survivors (many of them in their 20s), young abused children, and adolescents, in that order. I am intrigued by this because I have never consciously chosen to work less with adolescents, and yet I have never actively sought them out. Interestingly, that is just how things have worked out, and yet I know nothing occurs by accident. Writing this book has renewed my interest in working with adolescents: I have recently organized a group for adolescents with abuse-related issues, and I feel excited about starting it up. I have also told colleagues that I have openings in my caseload that I want to fill with adolescent clients.

I continue to feel optimistic about the potential for useful clinical interventions with abused adolescents, and I approach each case with hope. I also believe strongly in empowerment- or competency-based models, and feel that encouraging adolescents and helping them develop feelings of power, competency, and control is the greatest contribution I can make.

I have also learned that I cannot reach all youngsters I work with, no matter how dogged my efforts and how creative my style. I clearly remember some adolescents who terminated treatment abruptly, and for whom I could not make the therapy environment safe enough.

I worry about the youngsters I don't hear from, and often wonder how their lives turned out. I have been amazed by how often youngsters have written or tracked me down because they want to let me know how they are doing, or because they have something they want to discuss. I have been surprised (and delighted) by reading newspaper reports of a client who became a big football star in college, another youngster who became a probation officer, and another who became a successful cover-girl. I have also been distressed by news that a youngster I worked with was killed in the Gulf War, and two of my clients have died: one killed in a head-on collision, the other in a drive-by shooting.

Lastly, my sense is that when we become trusted allies and confidantes to adolescents, they repay us with great loyalty and respect. On two or three separate occasions, I feel that I have become a part of my young clients' extended family because I saw them throughout their latency and adolescence periods, and they felt that I cared for them, suspended judgment, advised them, didn't intentionally hurt them, and was "always there." What a privilege it has been to enter these lives in transition, and to make a contribution toward their growth.

References

Abidin, R. R. (1990). *Parenting stress index.* Charlotesville, VA: Pediatric Psychology Press.

Ainsworth, M. D. S., Blehar, N. C., Waters, E., & Wall, S. (1978). *Patterns of attachment: A psychological study of the Strange Situations.* Hillsdale, NJ: Erlbaum.

American Humane Association. (1978). *National analysis of official child abuse and neglect reporting.* Englewood, CO: Author. (Available from American Humane Association, 63 Inverness Drive East, Englewood, CO 80112-5117)

American Humane Association. (1986). *Highlights of official child neglect and abuse reporting.* Englewood, CO: Author. (Available from American Humane Association, 63 Inverness Drive East, Englewood, CO 80112-5117)

Ariès, P. (1960). *Centuries of childhood: A social history of family life* (R. Baldikc, Trans.). New York: Knopf, 1962.

Bagley, C. (1995). Early sexual experience and sexual victimization of children and adolescents. In G. A. Rekers (Ed.), *Handbook of child and adolescent sexual problems* (pp. 135–163). New York: Lexington Books.

Bandura, A., Ross, D., & Ross, S. (1961). Transmission of aggression through imitation of aggressive models. *Journal of Abnormal and Social Psychology, 63,* 575–582.

Bandura, A., & Walters, R. (1963). *Social learning and personality development.* New York: Holt, Rinehart & Winston.

Barbaree, H. E., Marshall, W. L., & Hudson, S. M. (Eds.). (1993). *The juvenile sex offender.* New York: Guilford Press.

Barker, P. (1990). *Clinical interviews with children and adolescents.* New York: Norton.

Barth, R. P., & Derezotes, D. S. (1990). *Preventing adolescent abuse: Effective intervention strategies and techniques.* New York: Lexington Books.

Bateson, G. (1980). *Mind and nature: A necessary unity.* Glasgow: Fontana/Collins.

Bean, B., & Bennett, S. (1993). *The me nobody knows: A guide for teen survivors.* Lexington, MA: Lexington Books.

Benedict, L. L. W., & Zantra, A. A. J. (1993). Family environmental characteristics as risk factors for childhood sexual abuse. *Journal of Clinical Child Psychology, 22,* 365–374.

Bloch, J. P. (1991). *Assessment and treatment of multiple personality and dissociative disorders.* Sarasota, FL: Professional Resource Exchange.

Blos, P. (1963). *On adolescence.* New York: Free Press.

Blos, P. (1967). The second individuation process of adolescence. *Psychoanalytic Study of the Child, 22,* 162–186.

Bowen, M. (1978). *Family theory in clinical practice.* New York: Jason Aronson.

Bowlby, J. (1969). *Attachment and loss: Vol. 1. Attachment.* New York: Basic Books.

Bowlby, J. (1973). *Attachment and loss: Vol. 2. Separation: Anxiety and anger.* New York: Basic Books.

Bowlby, J. (1988). *A secure base.* New York: Basic Books.

Boyer, D. (1995). Adolescent pregnancy: The role of sexual abuse. *National Resource Center on Child Sexual Abuse News, 4*(6), 1–3.

Boy's Town Press. (Producer). (1985). *Don't get stuck there* [Film]. (Available from Boy's Town Press, 13603 Flanagan Blvd., Boy's Town, NE 68010, 1-800-282-6657)

Briere, J. (1989). *Therapy for adults molested as children: Beyond survival.* New York: Springer.

Briere, J. (1992). *Child abuse trauma: Theory and treatment of the lasting effects.* Newbury Park, CA: Sage.

Briere, J., & Runtz, M. (1993). Childhood sexual abuse: Long-term sequelae and implications for psychological assessment. *Journal of Interpersonal Violence, 8,* 312–330.

Browne, A., & Finkelhor, D. (1986). Impact of child sexual abuse: A review of the literature. *Psychological Bulletin, 99,* 66–77.

Bukowski, W. N., Sippola, L., & Brender, W. (1993). Where does sexuality come from?: Normative sexuality from a developmental perspective. In H. E. Barbaree, W. L. Marshall, & S. M. Hudson (Eds.), *The juvenile sex offender* (pp. 84–103). New York: Guilford Press.

Burgess, A. W., & Hartman, C. R. (1995). Adolescent runaways and juvenile prostitution. In G. A. Rekers (Ed.), *Handbook of child and adolescent sexual problems* (pp. 187–209). New York: Lexington Books.

Burgess, A. W., Hartman, C. R., & McCormack, A. (1987). Abused to abuser: Antecedents of socially deviant behaviors. *American Journal of Psychiatry, 144,* 1431–1436.

Cantor, S. (1995). Inpatient treatment of adolescent survivors of sexual abuse. In M. Hunter (Ed.), *Child survivors and perpetrators of sexual abuse: Treatment innovations* (pp. 24–49). Newbury Park, CA: Sage.

Carnegie Council on Adolescent Development. (1995). *Great transitions: Preparing adolescents for a new century.* Washington, DC: Author.

Carrell, S. (1993). *Group exercises for adolescents: A manual for therapists.* Newbury Park, CA: Sage.

Chilman, C. (1983). *Adolescent sexuality in a changing society.* New York: Wiley.

Cicchetti, D., & Rizley, D. (1981). Developmental perspective on the etiology, intergenerational transmission, and sequelae of child maltreatment. *New Directions for Child Development, 11,* 31–55.

Cole, P. M., & Putnam, F. W. (1992). Effect of incest on self and social functioning: A developmental psychopathology perspective. *Journal of Consulting and Clinical Psychology, 60,* 174–184.

Coons, P. M. (1986). Psychiatric problems associated with child abuse: A review. In J. J. Jacobsen (Ed.), *Psychiatric sequelae of child abuse.* Springfield, IL: Charles C Thomas.

Coopersmith, S. (1967). *The antecedents of self-esteem.* San Francisco: W. H. Freeman.

Corder, B. F. (1994). *Structured adolescent psychotherapy groups.* Sarasota, FL: Professional Resources Press.

Courtois, C. A. (1979). Characteristics of a volunteer sample of adult women who experienced incest in childhood and adolescence. *Dissertation Abstracts International, 40A,* Nov.–Dec., 3194-A.

Courtois, C. A. (1988). *Healing the incest wound: Adult survivors in therapy.* New York: Norton.

Crain, W. (1992). *Theories of development: Concepts and applications* (3rd ed.). Englewood Cliffs, NJ: Prentice-Hall.

Cuffe, S. E., & Frick-Helms, S. B. (1995). Treatment interventions for child sexual abuse. In G. A. Rekers (Ed.), *Handbook of child and adolescent sexual problems* (pp. 232–251). New York: Lexington Books.

Culley, D. C., & Flanagan, C. H. (1995). Assessment of sexual problems in childhood and adolescence. In G. A. Rekers (Ed.), *Handbook of child and adolescent sexual problems* (pp. 14–30). New York: Lexington Books.

Delaney, J., Lupton, M., & Toth, E. (1988). *The curse: A cultural history of menstruation.* Urbana: University of Illinois Press.

Dolan, Y. (1991). *Resolving sexual abuse: Solution-focused therapy and Ericksonian hypnosis for adult survivors.* New York: Norton.

Donaldson, M. A., & Cordes-Green, S. (1994). *Group treatment of adult incest survivors.* Newbury Park, CA: Sage.

Durrant, M., & Kowalski, K. (1990). Overcoming the effects of sexual abuse. In M. Durrant & C. White (Eds.), *Ideas for therapy with sexual abuse* (pp. 65–110). (Available from the Dulwich Centre, Hutt Street, P.O. Box 7192, Adelaide, South Australia)

Durrant, M., & White, C. (Eds.). (1990). *Ideas for therapy with sexual abuse.*

(Available from the Dulwich Centre, Hutt Street, P.O. Box 7192, Adelaide, South Australia)

Edgcumbe, R., & Gavshon, A. (1985). Clinical comparisons of traumatic events and reactions. *Bulletin of the Anna Freud Center, 8,* 3–21.

Erikson, E. H. (1963). *Childhood and society* (2nd ed.). New York: Norton.

Farber, E. D., & Joseph, J. A. (1985). The maltreated adolescent: Patterns of physical abuse. *Child Abuse and Neglect, 9,* 201–206.

Finkelhor, D. (1995). The victimization of children: A developmental perspective. *American Journal of Orthopsychiatry, 65*(2), 177–193.

Finkelhor, D., & Berliner, L. (1995). Research on the treatment of sexually abused children: A review and recommendations. *Journal of American Academy of Child and Adolescent Psychiatry, 34*(11), 1408–1423.

Finkelhor, D., & Dziuba-Leatherman, J. (1994). Victimization of children. *American Psychologist, 49*(3), 173–183.

Finkelhor, D., Hotaling, G. T., & Sedlak, A. (1990). *Missing, abducted, runaway and throwaway children in America: First report.* Washington, DC: Juvenile Justice Clearinghouse.

Fisher, B., Berdie, J., Cook, J., & Day, N. (1980). *Adolescent abuse and neglect: Intervention strategies* (DHHS Publication No. 80-30266). Washington, DC: U.S. Government Printing Office.

Flannery, D. J., Torquati, J. C., & Lindemeier, L. (1994). The method and meaning of emotional expressions and experience during adolescence. *Journal of Adolescent Research, 9*(1), 8–27.

Forehand, R., & Wierson, M. (1993). The role of developmental factors in planning behavioral interventions for children: Disruptive behavior as an example. *Behavior Therapy, 24,* 117–141.

Freud, S. (1935). *A general introduction to psychoanalysis.* New York: Liveright.

Freud, S. (1954). *The origins of psychoanalysis: Letters to Wilhelm Fliess, notes and drafts.* New York: Basic.

Friedberg, R. D., Mason, C., & Fidaleo, M. D. (1992). *Switching channels: A cognitive-behavioral workbook for adolescents.* Odessa, FL: Psychological Assessment Resources.

Friedrich, W. N. (1995a). Managing disorders of self-regulation in sexually abused boys. In M. Hunter (Ed.), *Child survivors and perpetrators of sexual abuse: Treatment innovations* (pp. 3–23). Newbury Park, CA: Sage.

Friedrich, W. N. (1995b). *Psychotherapy with sexually abused boys: An integrated approach.* Newbury Park, CA: Sage.

Friedrich, W. N., Grambsch, P., Damon, L., Hewitt, S., Koverola, C., Lang, R., Wolfe, V., & Broghton, D. (1992). The Child Sexual Behavior Inventory: Normative and clinical contrast. *Psychological Assessment, 4,* 303–311.

Friedrich, W. N., Urquiza, A. J., & Beilke, R. L. (1986). Behavior problems in sexually abused young children. *Journal of Pediatric Psychology, 11,* 47–57.

Gagnon, J. H. (1972). The creation of the sexual in early adolescence. In J. Kagnon & R. Coles (Eds.), *Twelve to sixteen: Early adolescence* (pp. 231–257). New York: Norton.

Garbarino, J., Guttman, E., & Seeley, J. (1986). *The psychologically battered child.* San Francisco: Jossey-Bass.

"Generation excluded: A report chides America for neglecting adolescents." (1995, October 23). *Time,* p. 86.

Gerard, A. B. (1994). *Parent–child relationship inventory.* Los Angeles: Western Psychological Services.

Gil, E. (1988). *Treatment of adult survivors of childhood abuse.* Rockville, MD: Launch Press.

Gil, E. (1991). *The healing power of play: Working with abused children.* New York: Guilford Press.

Gil, E. (1995). *Systemic treatment of families who abuse.* San Francisco: Jossey-Bass.

Gil, E. (in press). *Slices and loaves: Working with children who dissociate.* Rockville, MD: Launch Press.

Gil, E., & Johnson, T. C. (1993). *Sexualized children: Assessment and treatment of sexualized children and children who molest.* Rockville, MD: Launch Press.

Gillis, J. (1981). *Youth and history: Tradition and change in European age relations.* New York: Academic Press.

Gomes-Schwartz, B., Horowitz, J., & Sauzier, M. (1985). Severity of emotional distress among sexually abused preschool, schoolage and adolescent children. *Hospital and Community Psychiatry, 36,* 503–508.

Haley, J. (1976). *Problem solving therapy.* San Francisco: Jossey-Bass.

Hart, L. E., Mader, L., Griffith, K., & deMendonca, M. (1989). Effects of sexual and physical abuse: A comparison of adolescent inpatients. *Child Psychiatry and Human Development, 20*(1), 49–57.

Hart, S. N., & Brassard, M. R. (1987). A major threat to children's mental health: Psychological maltreatment. *American Psychologist, 42,* 160–165.

Herman, J. (1992). *Trauma and recovery.* New York: Basic Books.

Hibbard, R. A., Ingersoll, G. M., & Orr, D. P. (1990). Behavioral risk, emotional risk, and child abuse among adolescents in a nonclinical setting. *Pediatrics, 86*(6), 896–901.

Hill, P. (1993). Recent advances in selected aspects of adolescent development. *Journal of Child Psychology & Psychiatry & Allied Professionals, 34*(1), 69–99.

Hussey, D., & Singer, M. I. (1993). Sexual and physical abuse: The Adolescent Sexual Concern Questionnaire. In M. I. Singer, L. T. Singer, & T. M. Anglin (Eds.), *Handbook for screening adolescents at psychosocial risk* (pp. 131–163). New York: Lexington Books.

Jaffee, P. G., Wolfe, D. A., & Wilson, S. K. (1990). *Children of battered women.* Newbury Park: Sage.

James, B. (1995). *Handbook for treatment of attachment-trauma problems in children.* New York: Lexington Books.

Janus, M. D., McCormack, A., Burgess, A. W., & Hartman, C. (1987). *Adolescent runaways: Causes and consequences.* Lexington, MA: Lexington Books.

Johnson, T. C. (1993). Childhood sexuality. In E. Gil & T. C. Johnson, *Sexualized children: Assessment and treatment of sexualized children and children who molest* (pp. 1–20). Rockville, MD: Launch Press.

Jones, D. P. H., & McGraw, J. M. (1987). Reliable and fictitious accounts of sexual abuse to children. *Journal of Interpersonal Violence, 2,* 27–45.

Jones, E. (1991). *Working with adult survivors of child sexual abuse.* (Systemic Thinking and Practice Series, Nos. 7–8). New York: Karnac Books.

Kamsler, A. (1990). Her-story in the making: Therapy with women who were sexually abused in childhood. In M. Durrant & C. White (Eds.), *Ideas for therapy with sexual abuse* (pp. 9–36). (Available from the Dulwich Centre, Hutt Street, P.O. Box 7192, Adelaide, South Australia)

Karen, R. (1994). *Becoming attached: Unfolding the mystery of the infant–mother bond and its impact on later life.* New York: Warner.

Katz, J. (1981, Spring). Social class in North American history. *Journal of Interdisciplinary History, 11.*

Kegan, R. (1982). *The evolving self.* Cambridge, MA: Harvard University Press.

Kendall-Tackett, K. A., Williams, L. M., & Finkelhor, D. (1993). Impact of sexual abuse on children: A review and synthesis of recent empirical studies. *Psychological Bulletin, 113*(1), 164–180.

Kluft, R. P. (1990). Incest and subsequent revictimization: The case of therapist–patient sexual exploitation, with a description of the sitting duck syndrome. In R. P. Kluft (Ed.), *Incest related syndromes of adult psychopathology* (pp. 263–287). Washington, DC: American Psychiatric Press.

Koff, E. (1983). Through the looking glass of menarche: What the adolescent girl sees. In S. Golub (Ed.), *Menarche* (pp. 77–86). New York: Lexington Books.

Kohlberg, L. (1981). *Essays on moral development: Vol. 1. The philosophy of moral development: Moral stages and the idea of justice.* San Francisco: Harper & Row.

Kolko, D. (1992). Characteristics of child victims of physical violence: Research findings and clinical implications. *Journal of Interpersonal Violence, 7,* 244–276.

Kramer, E. (1971). *Art as therapy with children.* New York: Schocken Books.

Krystal, H. (1978). Trauma and Affects. *Psychoanalytic Study of the Child, 33,* 81–116.

Linehan, M. M. (1993). *Skills training manual for treating borderline personality disorder.* New York: Guilford Press.

Linesch, D. G. (1988). *Adolescent art therapy.* New York: Brunner/Mazel.

Madanes, C. (1981). *Strategic family therapy.* San Francisco: Jossey-Bass.

Mann, L., Harmoni, R., & Power, C. (1989). Adolescent decision making: The development of competence. *Journal of Adolescence, 12,* 265–278.

Martinson, F. (1991). Normal sexual development in infancy and early childhood. In G. D. Ryan & S. L. Lane (Eds.), *Juvenile sexual offending: Causes, consequences, and correction* (pp. 57–82). New York: Lexington Books.

Mather, C. L., & Debye, K. (1994). *How long does it hurt?* San Francisco: Jossey-Bass.

McCann, L., Pearlman, L. A., Sakheim, D. K., & Abrahamson, D. J. (1988). Assessment and treatment of the adult survivor of childhood sexual abuse within a schema framework. In S. M. Sgroi (Ed.), *Vulnerable populations: Evaluation and treatment of sexually abused children and adult survivors* (pp. 77–102). New York: Lexington Books.

McDougall, J. (1982–1983). Alexithymia, psychosomatosis, and psychosis. *International Journal of Psychoanalytic and Psychotherapy, 9,* 379–388.

Merchant, D. A. (1990). *Treating abused adolescents: A program for providing individual and group therapy.* Holmes Beach, FL: Learning.

Minuchin, S. (1974). *Families and family therapy.* Cambridge, MA: Harvard University Press.

Moone, J. (1994). *Juvenile victimization: 1987–1992* (Fact Sheet 17). Washington DC: Office of Juvenile Justice and Delinquency Prevention, U.S. Department of Justice.

Moos, R. (1979). *Family environment scale.* Palo Alto, CA: Consulting Psychologists Press.

National Center for Health Statistics. (1995, July 11). *The Washington Post,* pp. 10–11.

Naumburg, M. (1987). *Dynamically oriented art therapy: Its principles and practice.* Chicago: Magnolia Street.

Newton, M. (1995). *Adolescence: Guiding youth through the perilous ordeal.* New York: Norton.

O'Hanlon, W. H., & Weiner-Davis, M. (1989). *In search of solutions: A new direction in psychotherapy.* New York: Norton.

Offer, D., & Sabshin, M. (1984). Adolescence: Empirical perspectives. In D. Offer & M. Sabshin (Eds.), *Normality and the life cycle* (pp. 76–107). New York: Basic Books.

Pearce, J. W., & Pezzot-Pearce, T. (1994). Attachment theory and its implications for psychotherapy with maltreated children. *Child Abuse and Neglect, 18*(5), 425–438.

Pelcovitz, D. (1984). Adolescent abuse: Family structure and implications for treatment. *Journal of the American Academy of Child Psychiatry, 23*(1), 85–90.

Perry, N. W. (1987). Child and adolescent development: A psycholegal perspective. In J. E. B. Myers (Ed.), *Child witness: Law and practice* (pp. 459–525). New York: Wiley.

Petersen, A., & Taylor, B. (1980). The biological approach to adolescence. In J. Adelson (Ed.), *Handbook of adolescent psychology.* New York: Wiley.

Piaget, J. (1970). *Structuralism.* New York: Harper & Row.

Piaget, J. (1971). *Psychology and epistemology: Toward a theory of knowledge.* New York: Viking.

Piaget, J. (1972). Intellectual evolution from adolescence to adulthood. *Human Development, 15,* 1–12.

Powers, J., & Eckenrode, J. (1992). *The epidemiology of adolescent maltreatment.* Paper presented at the Fourth Biennial Meeting, Society for Research on Adolescence, Washington, DC. (Distributed by Cornell University, Family Life Development Center, MVR Hall, Ithaca, NY 14853)

Putnam, F. W. (1990). Disturbances of "self" in victims of childhood sexual abuse. In R. P. Kluft (Ed.), *Incest related syndromes of adult psychopathology* (pp. 113–132). Washington, DC: American Psychiatric Press.

Putnam, F. W. (1991, October). *Behavioral and psychophysiological correlates of sexual abuse.* Paper presented at the Annual Meeting of the American Academy of Child and Adolescent Psychiatry, San Francisco.

Quinsey, V. L., Rice, M. E., Harris, G. T., & Reid, K. S. (1993). The phylogenetic and ontogenetic development of sexual age preferences in males: Conceptual and measurement issues. In H. E. Barbaree, W. L. Marshall, & S. M. Hudson (Eds.), *The juvenile sex offender* (pp. 143–163). New York: Guilford Press.

Rierdan, J., & Koff, E. (1980). The psychological impact of menarche: Integrative versus disruptive changes. *Journal of Youth and Adolescence, 9,* 49–58.

Rubin, J. A. (1984). *Child art therapy: Understanding and helping children grow* (rev. ed.). New York: Van Nostrand Reinhold.

Rubin, J. A. (Ed.). (1987). *Approaches to art therapy: Theory and technique.* New York: Brunner/Mazel.

Rutter, M., Graham, P., Chadwick, O., & Yule, W. (1976). Adolescent turmoil: Fact of fiction? *Journal of Child Psychology and Psychiatry, 17,* 35–56.

Ryan, G. (1991). The juvenile sex offender. In G. D. Ryan & S. L. Lane (Eds.), *Juvenile sexual offending: Causes, consequences, and correction* (pp. 143–160). New York: Lexington Books.

Sanford, L. T. (1990). *Strong at the broken places: Overcoming the trauma of childhood abuse.* New York: Avon Books.

Schetky, D. H. (1990). A review of the literature on the long-term effects of childhood abuse. In R. P. Kluft (Ed.), *Incest-related syndromes of adult psychopathology* (pp. 35–54). Washington DC: American Psychiatric Press.

Schofield, M. (1965). *The sexual behaviour of young people.* Boston: Little, Brown.

Schrodt, G., & Fitzgerald, B. (1987). Cognitive therapy with adolescents. *American Journal of Psychotherapy, XLI*(3), 402–408.

Selman, R. L., & Schultz, L. H. (1990). *Making a friend in youth: Developmental theory and pair therapy.* Chicago: University of Chicago Press.

Singer, M. I., Singer, L. T., & Anglin, T. M. (Eds.). (1993). *Handbook for screening adolescents at psychosocial risk.* New York: Lexington Books.

Smith, E. A. (1989). A biosocial model of adolescent sexual behavior. In G. R. Adams, R. Montemayor, & T. P. Gillotta (Eds.), *Biology of adolescent behavior and development* (pp. 143–167). Newbury Park, CA: Sage.

Smith, E. A., Udry, J., & Morris, N. M. (1985). Pubertal development and friends: A biosocial explanation of adolescent sexual behavior. *Journal of Health and Social Behavior, 26,* 183–192.

Sonkin, D. J. (1992). *Wounded boys, heroic men: A man's guide to recovering from child abuse.* Stamford, CT: Longmeadow Press.

Steen, C., & Monnette, B. (1989). *Treating adolescent sex offenders in the community.* Springfield, IL: Charles C Thomas.

Straus, M. A. (1994). *Beating the devil out of them: Corporal punishment in American families.* New York: Lexington Books.

Straus, M. B. (1988). Abused adolescents. In M. B. Straus (Ed.), *Abuse and victimization across the life span* (pp. 107–123). Baltimore: Johns Hopkins University Press.

Straus, M. B. (1994). *Violence in the lives of adolescents.* New York: Norton.

Terr, L. (1994). *Unchained memories: True stories of traumatic memories, lost and found.* New York: Basic Books.

Tobin-Richards, M. H., Boxer, A. M., & Petersen, A. C. (1983). The psychological significance of pubertal changes: Sex differences in perceptions of self during early adolescence. In J. Brooks-Gunn & A. Petersen (Eds.), *Girls at puberty* (pp. 127–177). New York: Plenum Press.

Trickett, P. K., & Putnam, F. W. (1993). Impact of child sexual abuse on females: Toward a developmental psychobiological integration. *Psychological Science, 4*(2), 81–87.

Ulman, E., & Dachinger, P. (Eds.). (1975). *Art therapy: In theory and practice.* New York: Schocken Books.

U.S. Department of Health and Human Services. (1995). *Child maltreatment 1993: Reports from the states to the National Center on Child Abuse and Neglect.* Washington, DC: U.S. Government Printing Office. (Available from the National Clearinghouse on Child Abuse and Neglect Information, P.O. Box 1182, Washington, DC 20013-1182)

van der Kolk, B. A. (Ed.). (1987). *Psychological trauma.* Washington, DC: American Psychiatric Press.

Vargas, L. A., & Koss-Chioino, J. D. (Eds.). (1992). *Working with culture: Psychotherapeutic interventions with ethnic minority children and adolescents.* San Francisco: Jossey-Bass.

Walsh, B. W., & Rosen, P. M. (1988). *Self-mutilation: Theory, research and treatment.* New York: Guilford Press.

Walt Disney Educational Productions. (Producer). (1985). *A time to tell* [Film]. (Available from Walt Disney Educational Productions, 105 Terry Drive, Suite 120, Newton, PA 18954, 1-800-295-5010)

Waterman, J., & Ben-Meir, S. (1993). Background literature. In J. Waterman, R. J. Kelly, M. K. Oliveri, & J. McCord, *Behind the playground walls: Sexual abuse in preschools* (pp. 11–29). New York: Guilford Press.

Waterman, J., & Kelly, R. J. (1993). Mediators of effects on children: What enhances optimal functioning and promotes healing? In J. Waterman, R. J. Kelly, M. K. Oliveri, & J. McCord, *Behind the playground walls: Sexual abuse in preschools* (pp. 222–239). New York: Guilford Press.

Wauchope, B., & Straus, M. A. (1990). Physical punishment and physical abuse of American children: Incidence rates by age, gender, and occupational class. In M. A. Straus & R. J. Gelles (Eds.), *Physical violence in American families: Risk factors and adaptations to violence in 8,145 families.* New Brunswick, NJ: Transaction.

Weiner, I., & Elkind, D. (1972). *Child development: A core approach.* New York: Wiley.

Westen, D. (1994). The impact of sexual abuse on self structure. In D. Cicchetti & S. L. Toth (Eds.), *Disorders and dysfunctions of the self* (pp. 223–249). Rochester, NY: University of Rochester Press.

White, M., & Epston, D. (1990). *Narrative means to therapeutic ends.* New York: Norton.

Wolfe, D. A. (1987). *Child abuse: Implications for child development and psychopathology.* Newbury Park, CA: Sage.

Young, K. R., West, R. P., Smith, D. J., & Morgan, D. P. (1994). *Teaching self-management strategies to adolescents.* Longmont, CO: Sopris West.

Zarb, J. M. (1992). *Cognitive-behavioral assessment and therapy with adolescents.* New York: Brunner/Mazel.

Index